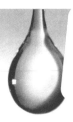

# WELLNESS
## OUR BIRTHRIGHT
### How to Give a Baby the
### Best Start for Life

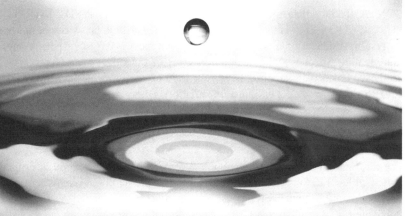

## Vivien Clere Green

LIFESUCCESS PUBLISHING, LLC
8900 E Pinnacle Peak Road, Suite D240
Scottsdale, AZ  85255

| Telephone: | 800.473.7134 |
| Fax: | 480.661.1014 |

| E-mail: | admin@lifesuccesspublishing.com |
| ISBN: | 1-59930-020-6 |
| Cover: | Patti Knoles & LifeSuccess Publishing |
| Layout: | Lloyd Arbour & LifeSuccess Publishing |

COMPANIES, ORGANIZATIONS, INSTITUTIONS, AND INDUSTRY PUBLICATIONS: Quantity discounts are available on bulk purchases of this book for reselling, educational purposes, subscription incentives, gifts, sponsorship, or fundraising. Special books or book excerpts can also be created to fit specific needs such as private labeling with your logo on the cover and a message from a VIP printed inside. For more information please contact our Special Sales Department at LifeSuccess Publishing.

## Medical Disclaimer

The information contained in this book is provided for your general information only. Neither LifeSuccess Publishing, LLC nor the author, Vivien Clere Green provide medical advice or engage in the practice of medicine. LifeSuccess Publishing, LLC and Vivien Clere Green do not recommend particular medical treatments for any individual. For questions regarding your medical condition LifeSuccess Publishing, LLC and Vivien Clere Green recommend that you consult your physician or health care professional before pursuing any course of treatment.

"An inspiring, practical book that simplifies the physical and emotional journey of wellness and pregnancy."

**Stuart Korth, DO, DPO**
Co-Founder and Director of Osteopathy
at the Osteopathic Centre for Children


"Human beings have difficult births compared with other mammals, but Nature has found solutions to overcome these handicaps. Read Vivien Clere Green's illuminating book, Wellness Our Birthright, to discover these solutions for yourself. This is a comprehensive but easy to read guide written for the general public."

**Dr Michel Odent**
Director of Primal Health Research,
Obstetrician, Visionary, Author of *The Caesarian*


"It is becoming ever clearer that a number of very serious diseases, like cancer and a weakened immune system are being generated in our children before they are even born. Vivien's work sheds light on how we can attempt to prevent this. Sadly, ignorance of the latest research and knowledge abounds. This book goes a long way in attempting to correct this."

**Chris Woollams MA (Oxon)**
Co-Founder of CANCERactive
Author of *Everything You Need to Know to Help You Beat Cancer*


"It is a great pleasure to endorse Vivien Clere Green's book. For many years Vivien has been practising as a natural health consultant as well as basing her own and her family's life on the same principles. Vivien walks the walk as well as talking the talk. The issues raised in this book are optimistic and its emphasis is very much on eating well, exercising and having an optimistic outlook to birth and parenting. I enjoyed reading the book".

**Dr. Yehudi Gordon**
Obstetrician, Gynaecologist, Author and
Pioneer of informed choice and integrated healthcare.
Author of *Birth and Beyond*


"Anaesthetic is made out to be the magic bullet, the long term after effects can be devastating, as it proved to be for me. "

**Mrs Kathleen Ford**
Mother, Florida

"Vivien's writing is thoughtful, loving, and tender. She focuses on birth and parenting with sensitivity and awareness."

**Sheila Kitzinger**
noted authority on pregnancy and childbirth,
awarded the MBE for her services to education for childbirth
Author of *Birth Crisis*


"Once in a while someone appears who makes total sense of everything they say ~ in language we can all understand. Wellness Our Birthright may become the bible for every mother who wants the very best for her child."

**Larry Brooks**
Entrepreneur and Coach


"I challenge you to find anyone as youthful in spirit or body as Vivien - after bringing up five gorgeous, healthy, children. She is learned in many disciplines and inspires me daily."

**Neroli Lacey**
Journalist and Writer


"Vivien Clere Green in Wellness Our Birthright helps people manage the world's number one cause of physical, mental & emotional pain in life: it's called fear. I applaud her in helping to move people to a belief in their higher spiritual self, a place where neither fear nor limits exist."

**John Kanary**
Life Coach
Author of *Breaking through Limitations*


"A very much needed book that I feel confident to recommend as a Pilates teacher, it offers accurate information and sound advice in an easy to read format. It couldn't have come at a better time for me personally!"

**Claire Dinsdale**
Pilates Teacher, Oxfordshire


"The birth of my second daughter, Freya, was so much more than I ever imagined I could achieve. This was in no small part due to Vivien being a part of it. She gave both my husband and myself, the confidence to make the "home birth" choice and she helped me to believe in the wonderful capabilities of the female body and find that potential in myself"

**Libby Chant**
Mother, England

"Vivien has successfully shared the fruits of her extensive research and experiences as a practitioner and radiantly positive mother. This complete guide gives you the confidence to make knowledgeable decisions and help avoid some of the common pitfalls that so many women encounter. Wellness our Birthright is not only for mothers to be, but is for anyone interested in health and well-being. Vivien promotes a long term and sustainable approach to increasing our own wellness and most importantly, for the health of the next generation."

**Monica Byant BSc.(Hons)**
International Health Writer and Educator

"I truly feel privileged to endorse Vivien Clere Green's book Wellness Our Birthright! As a naturopathic doctor and psychologist, I have witnessed women of all ages struggle with their anxieties and fear in times of pregnancy.

It is my conviction that women possess the innate ability to enjoy effortless pregnancy if they work in harmony with nature to have a natural childbirth. Vivien's book gently takes every pregnant woman and mothers by the hand, encouraging them to comply with nature, the way it should be!"

**Olakunbi Korostensky ND / MA**
Founder and CEO of Awaken Women International.
A community which encourages women around the world to fully embrace their spiritual strengths as a natural way of being.

"Having had so many difficulties conceiving, the joy of giving birth to two wonderful children is miraculous. Vivien's help and guidance changed mine and my husband's lives. How special it is to have all this help in written form in her book Wellness our Birthright. Thank you!"

**Joanna Blythe**
Mother, London

Every time I hear someone talking about the benefits of natural birth, I feel a pang of sadness – I did not know about the long term advantages including improved immunity for the baby. I wish I had known what I do now as I wouldn't have chosen an elective caesarean. Vivien makes it very clear in her book *Wellness our Birthright*, a **must** read.

**Josefa Gonzalez**
Mother and Photographer

*"I honour, with love and gratitude,*
*all mothers from the beginning of time."*

# Contents

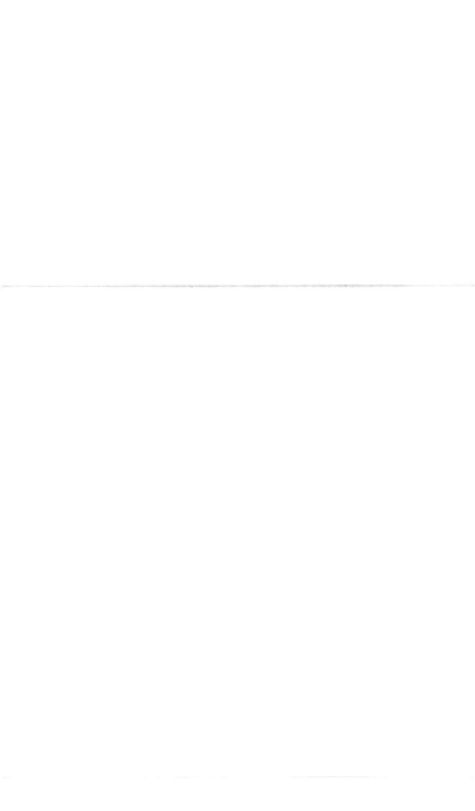

# A *huge thank you to everyone who has helped me with this book*

Special thanks goes first to my family, my husband Richard and my children Sophie, William, Alexander, Francesca and Alicia for all their valuable contributions, continued support, patience and love, and without whom none of this could have come about in the first place; to my sister, Caroline Cary, whose continued encouragement helped me to achieve this; to Trudi Clay for her wisdom, to Chris Woollams, whose unhesitating and generous help made the book happen; to Justine Lawrence, my wonderful assistant whose inspiration and perseverance has been unequalled; to Michel Odent who "opened the door to me" and for his Doula information sessions; to Stuart Korth who has helped all my children; to Martine Faure Alderson who told me "there was work to be done"; to Larry Brooks, for his inspiration and never failing support; to Claire, my gifted pilates teacher, to John Kanary, who helped me not only set the goal but gave me the belief that I could achieve it and who also put me in touch with an amazing man, Gerry Robert.

A huge thank you goes to Gerry and his awesome team at LifeSuccess Publishing - my project manager, Kandi Miller, designer, Patti Knoles and editor, Angi Eagleton. To my exceptional Obstetricians: Yehudi Gordon, who was there at the beginning of my personal journey and Mark Charnock who was there at the end; to my fantastic midwives, especially, Gwen Attwood and to all friends and colleagues who have helped me along the way. Thanks to all at Neways, Biopathica, Ainsworth, Biocare and to all my wonderful patients, babies and children in the practice.

**Finally, a huge thank you goes to you the reader for making this whole mission worthwhile.**

# *Foreword*

With decades of clinical experience, both my colleagues and I have seen, over and over again, babies, children and mothers who suffer from traumas and strains received as a result of birth. Paediatric Osteopathy offers a non-invasive system of natural medicine using gentle techniques to rebalance the problems within the body's systems. Although in many instances we have very encouraging results, how much better it would be if these traumas could be avoided in the first place. Prevention is better than cure.

Today, what we need more than ever, in an impatient society looking for instant results and paying no heed to the long term consequences of our actions, is accurate knowledge and sound advice to help us on the way. Here is such knowledge and advice written clearly in language everyone can understand.

This book looks at the health and well-being of the parents themselves, starting from even before conception and takes the reader through the steps of pregnancy, birth, breastfeeding and early motherhood. The reader gains insight to the profound effect that these steps have on the baby for its entire life and the importance of creating a healthy environment, physically, mentally and emotionally all the way though. Mothers and Fathers can look at birth as a natural physiological event, not an illness, where so-called modern methods should stay in the background and allow the natural processes to take place.

In this book, Vivien goes a long way to clear up all the mixed messages and unnecessary fear which is often intensified by the media, television and newspapers, so that women not only approach pregnancy with ease but have the trust and confidence in the natural birthing process.

**Stuart Korth DO, DPO**
- Director of Osteopathy at The OCC
(The Osteopathic Centre for Children)

# Imagine...

Imagine that either you, someone you know, someone in your family or a professional colleague, are going to have a baby. Wouldn't you want to ensure that they are well informed for this journey? Wouldn't you want to make this experience wonderful, to give this new baby the best possible start in life? To set patterns for this baby to be a healthier, happier as well as a loving and caring human being? That is exactly what this book offers - accurate information and guidance compiled from both personal and professional experiences, as well as extensive research and studies, to help all those on this journey.

A woman's body is designed by nature with a built-in genetic blueprint to reproduce, to give birth and to nurture new life, thus ensuring survival of the race as we have through countless eons of time. Down through the ages we have gathered experiences and if we raise our awareness and put this knowledge and wisdom to good use, we can make this journey not only easier and better for all concerned but one full of joy and happiness.

So many choices are open to us. So much information and so many opinions are available that it is challenging to steer a clear path. Armed with knowledge, we can help avoid some of the needless suffering and missed opportunities. One thing that we have known instinctively for centuries and is now being proven by science is that the way we nurture our unborn babies and welcome them into the world has a profound effect on them for the rest of their lives.

Keep an open mind and don't be surprised by information that challenges your ways of thinking, we have a job to do: make Wellness our birthright. As Suzanne Arms, renowned author, photographer and speaker in this field, says so beautifully:

"If we hope to create a non-violent world where respect and kindness replace fear and hatred, we must begin with how we treat each other at the beginning of life. For that is where our deepest patterns are set. From these roots grow fear and alienation or love and trust."

I was fortunate to have such information as I started my own journey some twenty-five years ago. Being a Natural Health Consultant and Practitioner, I knew to eat a wholesome diet and I combed the health food shops for organically grown foods (not then readily available). I also researched the various options for childbirth. When unsure, I always looked for ways to work with my genetic blueprint, an attempt to understand the natural laws. I followed advice from those who had experienced natural birth themselves or from professionals who assisted others in this way. Like many people at this stage, I had not a clue about pregnancy or birth; perhaps more unusually, I had never even held a newborn baby. I am the eldest of a small family. Both of my parents were only children, so there were no aunts, uncles or cousins.

When I became pregnant, home pregnancy tests were insufficiently reliable and I had to take a urine sample to my local surgery and wait for nearly 10 days for the results. So my journey began. An appointment was duly made with the gynaecologist and when I asked about being in an upright position for birth, he seemed disapproving, saying it was rather difficult to monitor the baby's heartbeat. I came away with a sense of helplessness. So I went to see another, Yehudi Gordon, who had a completely different attitude. In fact, he not only encouraged women to be upright and go for natural birth, he took the lead and is well renowned in this field.

Gradually all the pieces fell into place. I started yoga, went to antenatal (prenatal) classes, saw other women both pregnant and breastfeeding, held a newborn baby and witnessed baby massage. My tummy grew bigger and bigger and finally the day arrived and my contractions started. I put my hand on my tummy thinking of the little person inside, wondering how it was going to come out. One thing I knew for certain: I had already made my up mind that I was going for a natural birth and nothing was going to put me off. It was with this attitude that I went through the birth. I switched off completely, went into my own world and my body's ancient genetic coding came into action. Some hours later, I delivered Sophie, a 7.4lb baby girl. I did it without any painkillers or medical intervention whatsoever. I was euphoric.

Breastfeeding fell into place easily with the inevitable trials and tribulations and mixed emotions of euphoria, disbelief and tiredness. But I never imagined the love that I would feel for this tiny, miraculous little bundle.

As my baby girl, Sophie, grew, I weaned her and then continued with my studies and trainings in holistic health, often leaving my husband to fend for himself at the weekend with this new delight in his life. My practice grew with special emphasis on helping women with infertility, pregnancy and motherhood problems. I subsequently went on to have two more children naturally and I then suffered an ordeal, which nearly led to my womb being removed (a hysterectomy) and would more than likely have left me infertile.

So imagine how surprised I felt when, in my early forties, I found that I was, not only pregnant again but, expecting twins! What joy! However, now I found myself in the high-risk category with the expectation that these babies would be delivered by elective caesarean. With all my research, clinical experience and training as a Natural Health Professional, this was not what I wanted. Indeed as a Registered Member of the British Institute for Complementary Medicine, using bio-regulatory medicine, I felt I owed it not only to myself and my patients but also to women generally, to practice what I preach. It took a few attempts to find a gynaecologist who was open to my having a natural birth. I have to confess that, on my first visit, I did break down saying that I knew I had the capacity to give birth naturally to a single baby but did not know how I would manage two. Very reassuringly, he said: "It is only one labour and two pushes." I knew then that I could do it.

Nine months later, I was blessed with two beautiful baby girls, Francesca, 6lbs 12ozs and Alicia, 6lbs 2ozs. I delivered them naturally, at term, without any intervention whatsoever and I established breastfeeding very quickly. I then went on to feed them exclusively on my breast milk for six months before introducing solids to their diets. The Wellness Action Plan Programme worked for me again!

Not long afterwards, I took the babies for a check up with a close colleague and friend, a Naturopath and Acupuncturist. According to her assessment, she was delighted with the health of the babies and with my quick recovery. She looked at me and said: "Vivien, you have had the good fortune to have knowledge to help you achieve all this." She continued "You need to share this with others so that they can be as fortunate, too. Maybe you should write a book."

So, the first seed about writing this book was planted in my mind. I was then further inspired by all the experiences in my own practice with helping women, not only with fertility challenges but also with all the complications through pregnancy and the early stages of motherhood. I felt that some of their suffering could have been avoided had they known certain things in advance. Equally, a number of cases had tremendous joy and happiness through their experiences, many of whom kindly gave me permission to write up their personal stories (case histories). This was further endorsed by results from an independent study that I carried out on childbirth. I share these experiences with you, the reader, as with others in the practice in order that we may gain insight and understanding that can make your life or someone else's easier.

When enough people are inspired by what they read here to help spread the word, we will indeed raise healthier and happier children and so help not only the present generation but future ones, too.

# The Beginning

Suddenly there was an explosion! The earth had moved! Streams and sparks of coloured light were flying everywhere, all colours of the rainbow. It was like sunlight shining through crystal. Two microscopic cells united. One was squiggly, soft and round and the other was even smaller and tadpole-like; it was this latter one which succeeded in penetrating the barrier. The beginning of life as we know it on this planet earth has begun and the secret genetic code has been unlocked. Rapid cell division takes place, forming a new embryo and placenta, all encapsulated in the wonderful cocoon of its mother.

Just imagine, you are this new embryo, only a few days old. What would it be like? Well, let your imagination roam. You are just about to begin a journey of such a story.

I, this newly formed and rapidly growing being, have a sense, not a defined one yet, but just a sense of floating in liquid. Gradually over the weeks, I become more and more aware of this liquid. It is lovely. I just float around, sometimes the water is relatively still with just the odd ripple here and there and at other times, the movement is so rapid that I am constantly moving. I aim to find a balanced spot! Usually there is a constant reassuring rhythm, it changes intensity and pace, just as the sea can be calm with gentle lapping waves. When all of a sudden the pace changes, a wind starts blowing and the movement changes to rapid, crashing waves or, in my case, ripples.

I am aware that there is another rhythm developing, a much faster one. I later learn that this is my heartbeat and I am five weeks old.

More and more cells divide and the weeks go by. And as this happens I find I can roll around and somersault. What fun I am having! This liquid doesn't just surround me, it goes in and out of my lungs and I can even swallow it too!

There seems to be a pattern of stillness and quiet and then movement and action. Could this be night and day? So much is unknown to me. I am now sixteen weeks old and I can touch around my mouth, I feel movements in my body.

Now something is changing, I can hear rumbling and gurgling, which cause more ripples. Did I say hear? Yes! I can hear now. There are so many different sounds and echoes within the never-ending rumblings of the intestines.

All sorts of exciting things are happening to me – I can taste too! The water tastes salty and I have just worked out that the object that keeps going past my mouth is lovely to suck on, it is my thumb. Oh well! Time for more somersaults and roly-poly's.

Weeks go by and I constantly grow bigger and bigger. And as I do, I make more and more discoveries. Would you believe it now I can play a grabbing game with a long stringy pipe, which you know as my Mother's umbilical cord? As it brushes past my face, I reach out to touch it. Sometimes I miss and then I move again and lose it. The best is when I succeed in holding it so that I pull it towards me turning me upside down.

What a beautiful sound! Let me hear more! It is my mother singing. The water is rippling and the colours inside here are amazing. I have never seen colours like this before! I've only just felt them. Ah! My mother's voice, I am constantly aware of it, I know all the different tones and rhythms. When she is stressed or angry, it's not very comfortable at all, I am just hurled from one side to the other. It is a huge relief when it's over! Now this lovely sound of her singing makes me feel safe and secure. I hope she never stops. When she does, I just keep waiting for her to start again. I think it makes me grow! Just listening to her speaking is special. You see, as she breathes and moves her muscles it makes different patterns in the water, sometimes jerky, sometimes smooth and calm. It just depends on what she is saying.

The constant noises inside are my heartbeat, my mother's heartbeat and her digestive juices, which can be very loud sometimes. When she drinks water, I hear a cascade of gurglings.

At night when my mother sleeps, it is so quiet and spacious that I can move about easily! In the morning, she massages her tummy with some oil that has a tangerine smell. I move nearer to her hand and if I am asleep, I wake up and turn to look at the colours coming from her hand. You see, her touch creates colours inside my dark, red world. I am already twenty-six weeks old and my eyes are open. If I hear a sudden noise, it makes my heart race.

I am growing very big now and there is not so much movement. I can't play the somersault games any more, but I can dream now and even process some of my first memories. I have a regular pattern of waking and sleeping and sometimes I love to stretch my legs and give a good kick. I play a game with my mother - when I kick, she touches my foot and then I kick again. We wait for each other to play this game. She usually does it when she is lying down and I have more space then.

Oh, what is that bright light? I do wish people out there knew how sensitive I am. I hate loud banging noise and bright lights. I do love music. My mother talks about Mozart or Beethoven, whatever that is, but it is good when you are inside like I am.

I am coming up to the last week, I believe, or that is what I hear said on the outside. I am ready to see the outside world. So I have started to wriggle down and find a good position.

Now it is time for the dance to begin. I just had a message from my mother's body that she is ready and my lungs have just sent a message to hers saying they are ready. So I start by tapping my head on her cervix. This is at the bottom of her womb and it needs to open up to let me out.

I am feeling pressure on the outside of my mother's tummy and squeezing movements from her muscles. I am being massaged and very gently I wriggle further and further down. Then there is a pause and I find a comfortable position and wait. Very soon the squeezing movements start again and I wriggle even further down. Everything stops and there is a lull again. This pattern continues for a long time. As the squeezing movements intensify, I rotate until I can glimpse a little bit of light creeping in, so the hole must be opening.

My mother is making deep moaning noises, very soothing. This goes on for some time and then my skull bones slide across as I am pushed through this lovely warm tunnel. It is the best feeling I have had yet, so tight and snug.

Now I am being pushed in and out in an intense rhythm. My body is wriggling further down and I can see the light. With a whoosh I am sliding down and after a moment's pause my head pops out. Then with a gush, my body and all the water I have been immersed in comes out into the new world with me.

It is freezing out here! A hand lifts me onto my mother's skin, which is so warm and soft and as I root around, I find her nipple and suck on it. Then I look around and everything is dark and hazy until I see my mother's eyes. They are pools of light. I cannot take mine off hers; they are so incredible. I cannot bear to close mine in case they disappear. No, they haven't gone away, she is still looking at me. She smells lovely too! I reach up with my hand and touch her breast and we lie there in blissful contentment. I am born.

*"I best take care of my body.*
*Where else would I live?"*

**Yobe Komada**

. . . especially now there are two of us sharing it!

# *The 6 Steps*

Congratulations! You have made a decision – a decision to become a mother. Indeed, you may already be a mother, or on the way to becoming a mother again, or you may be in a position to help someone who is. What type of mother do you want to be? Do you want to enjoy the whole experience? How do you want to look afterwards? Now imagine you are that new baby. How would you want your mother to be - healthy, happy, full of positive emotion? Or ill, angry, depressed, full of negativity and toxins? It is said that a baby's number one wish is to choose its parents wisely! So let's take a look at how we might be able to increase those chances of you giving your baby the best start and also of you being the best mother possible.

This book looks first at the foundations for achieving the best possible health that you can: Wellness. I have called it *The Wellness Action Plan*. This requires an understanding of what is needed to create a healthy lifestyle both physically and mentally. This Plan is applicable all the way through life including pregnancy and the various stages of motherhood. In the subsequent chapters, we will focus on the specific advice for each stage: pre-pregnancy, pregnancy, birth, the critical hour after birth and breastfeeding. I have also included case histories and stories from my practice, my research and from my own life illustrate the Wellness concept.

*STEP 1* lays out the strategy and outlines an action plan to achieve Wellness. It covers what we need to eat and drink, a wholesome diet, the importance of taking nutritional supplements, having good dental, spinal and muscular health, exercising, removing harmful ingredients and toxins, as well as eliminating bad habits and how we think. This is applicable to anyone of any age.

*STEP 2* is what needs to be done in addition to the Wellness Action Plan before conception by both the prospective mother and father to ensure the best for the babies as yet unconceived. It is absolutely essential that both parents, but especially the mother, are in good health before starting on this journey. Preparation should, ideally, start a minimum of six months prior to conception.

*STEP 3* covers pregnancy. If you want the seed to grow to a healthy plant, it needs the right conditions, the right minerals, the right amount of water and the right environment. So it is with pregnancy.

*STEP 4* is about the actual birth. The changing physiology of the mother, trusting in her body and mind to experience childbirth as nature intended. How a baby is born has life-long consequences and the birth affects the baby's behaviour and health for its entire adult life.

*STEP 5* the "Critical Hour" refers to the time immediately after birth. It is vital during this hour for the mother and baby to be undisturbed so that they can bond - fall in love, so to speak - and breastfeeding can begin. Breast milk is nature's elixir for the baby with its own health giving properties and emotionally related consequences.

*STEP 6* offers tips and guidance for after the baby is born. It looks at essential guidelines for both the mother and baby for breastfeeding and some of the most important practices that will help give the baby the best wellness possible.

# *Step 1 - Achieving Wellness*

Wellness is radiant physical and mental health. It is a priceless commodity that is not simply the absence of illness, aches and pains, constant sniffles, depression and chronic illness. It is the sort of health that makes you feel wonderful, vibrant, like a million dollars, full of energy and ready to bounce out of bed in the mornings knowing that you are in tip top form with a properly functioning immune system. However, we are inclined to take our health for granted and expect it to be our birthright, but Wellness does not just happen. It has to be nurtured and maintained. In other words, Wellness needs to be an actively pursued goal.

Most of us do have the raw materials, but it is up to us whether we cultivate them or not. This first chapter, the Wellness Action Plan, goes through the necessary steps to achieve Wellness. It covers what we need to eat and drink, a wholesome diet, the importance of taking nutritional supplements, having good dental, spinal and muscular health, exercising, removing harmful ingredients and toxins, as well as eliminating bad habits such as smoking, drinking and even how we think. We also have to learn to look for early symptoms of imbalance such as headaches, indigestion, allergies, constipation, poor circulation, excess weight and learn to rectify these both physically and mentally.

I believe that everyone has the right to know how to achieve Wellness for not only themselves but for the next generation, too. It will have a knock on effect, just like a line of dominos. As one generation improves its health so can the next and so on.

## The Wellness Action Plan

To achieve Wellness, we have to understand how our bodies and minds work, they work together. Many of us are familiar with the phrase "we are what we eat" but perhaps not so familiar with "we are what we think." How does this help us? After all, it is not as if we can just stop thinking like we can abstain from food. Is it? No, this is true, but with current knowledge, we can use our thinking to enhance our lives. A tremendous amount of work has been done to understand the power of thought, especially in sports psychology. Athletes use their minds to reach goals and targets that push their bodies beyond known boundaries. So let us use some of this current understanding of the power of thought to help us achieve Wellness.

Science and theology, two opposite approaches to life, both agree that there is an infinite power that works in us, through us and all around us. The scientists call it energy and the theologians call it God. So for the sake of argument here, I have called it "spirit." We are spiritual beings with an intellect housed in a physical body. Our mind has two parts to our intellect, a conscious and sub-conscious. The difference between the two is that the conscious mind has the ability to either accept or reject an idea it receives, whereas the subconscious cannot. It will accept everything as being true irrespective of whether the idea is positive or negative. Conscious thoughts when attached to feelings will automatically filter through to the subconscious where they are stored. This builds belief systems (often a jumble of positive and negative ones), of who we are and what we are

14

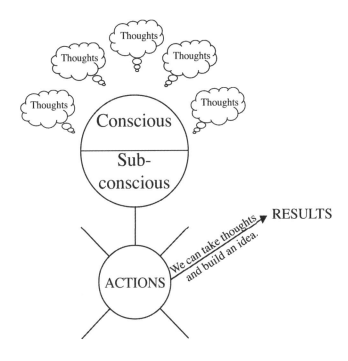

about and will govern our actions, which in turn produces our results. It is how we act and what we do that leads to our results. Now, if we try to alter our results by our actions alone, we will not be successful because we need to incorporate our thinking processes and our feelings to do so.

The challenge is that we measure every new idea by our existing belief systems (paradigms) that are built in to our subconscious, if the idea does not meet our paradigm we reject it instead of re-evaluating our belief systems. Let me give you a really good example: You have an idea to have a baby. Your belief/paradigm is "giving birth is going to hurt." How do you know? Does it have to? Then you say: "I'm going to need painkillers, anything to avoid the pain." Are you sure? Where did this information come from? Was it someone with wisdom and knowledge, or was it just someone's opinion? Have you considered what the long-term effects may be of using painkillers? And so it goes on.

The best bet is to keep an open mind, gain knowledge on the subject, ask those who are experienced or collect opinions from those you admire and respect in the field and then challenge some of these in built beliefs or paradigms. This book may do this for you as you read things that do not fit your existing paradigm, so do not be tempted to reject this information out of hand. I would ask you to keep an open mind.

*"The mind is like a parachute, it works best when open."*

**Larry Brooks**

## What should I eat?

We can't get away from it. "You are what you eat and absorb." The key is to provide the body with the best food possible so that every cell has what it needs. For this to happen, there must be a balance of good quality proteins, unrefined carbohydrates, unsaturated fats and plenty of organically grown fruit and vegetables.

Buy organically grown produce to avoid harmful pesticides and artificial chemicals. More than 25 million tons of pesticides are used each year in the UK and residues are found on nearly half of all fruit and vegetables tested. Sometimes there are up to seven different compounds and these compounds are believed to be even more toxic. Many pesticides are known or suspected to be hormone disrupters, which means that they interfere with the chemical messaging system in the body. They cause brain dysfunction, memory loss, heart problems, birth defects and the US Environmental Protection Agency states that pesticide residues are among the top three environmental cancer risks.

| What's best to eat? | Why? |
|---|---|
| **Vegetables** | |
| Eat plenty of these, organically grown, at each meal.<br><br>Always eat green and high coloured vegetables such as red peppers, carrots, sweet potatoes. | Reduces exposure to harmful pesticides and artificial chemicals. They are very alkalising and contain many nutrients: antioxidants, minerals, carotenoids, lycopenes, flavenoids and fibre. |
| **Fruits** | |
| Contrary to popular belief, raw fruit is better eaten before the meal, organically grown and ripe.<br><br>Eat dark coloured fruits such as blueberries, blackberries, cherries. | Very cleansing and alkalising, contains antioxidants, minerals, carotenoids, lycopenes, flavenoids and fibre. If eaten after a meal, fruit can cause fermentation in the stomach and should be avoided. |
| **Proteins** | |
| Fish – eat at least twice weekly. | Very good for you, especially oily fish like organic salmon, sardines, mackerel and herring, which contain fish oils known as Omega 3. |
| Meat - only eat from animals reared organically or to a very high standard. Use meat stocks. | This will be free from harmful hormonal and medicinal substances. |
| Eggs - use those from free range and organically reared hens. | Any animal that is fed as closely as possible to the natural laws will be healthier, free of toxic ingredients and hormones. |

| What's best to eat? | Why? |
| --- | --- |
| **Vegetarian proteins** | |
| Tofu and soya (soy) products, combine lentils with nuts or grains.<br><br>Essential to combine grains and pulses/nuts/seeds so that all the amino acids are ingested at the same time. | |
| **Essential Fats** | |
| To be clear, there are good and bad fats. In order for minerals, vitamins and nutrients to be absorbed into the cells, the essential fats are needed to "open the door". The bad fats do the complete opposite, they block this process.<br><br>As a bonus, essential fats help you feel satisfied after eating.<br><br>There is an old wives' tale that says women who have had babies are less brainy! Well, there is an element of truth. If the pregnant mother doesn't get enough of these essential fats, the baby will take her mother's supply and reserves, some of which come from her brain! So have enough and both you and your baby will be brighter! | |
| Fresh nuts such as almonds, brazils, hazelnuts and walnuts - and seeds such as sunflower, pumpkin, sesame, hemp and flax. | In order for a baby to grow, it needs essential fatty acids, which cannot be made in the body but can be obtained from these food sources.<br><br>These can be eaten whole, or as un-refined, cold pressed oil.<br><br>Note: use these for salad dressings or added to food after cooking – but NOT for cooking as they are unstable and turn into a "bad" fat. |
| Cold pressed, un-refined olive oil and coconut butter. | Only cook with olive oil or coconut butter as they are more stable when heated which means they do not cause damage to the body. |
| Butter from grass-fed, organically reared animals. | Higher content of nutrients and reduced risk of hormones and chemicals. |

| What's best to eat? | Why? |
|---|---|
| **Carbohydrates** | |
| Wholegrains should be unrefined: barley, rye, oats (porridge), buckwheat, millet and quinoa. | Processing removes much of the valuable nutrition and fibre. |
| Wholemeal bread. Wholemeal, un-refined flours such as spelt, rye, buckwheat and wholewheat. | White flour is devoid of the wheat germ (internal food supply of the seed enabling it to grow) and the endosperm (the outside of the grain providing roughage). The wheat germ is the most nutritious ingredient in wholemeal flour, but due to its short shelf life, manufacturers remove it so that their products will have a longer shelf life.<br><br>Wholemeal, dense, bread is better. The light airy type has a much higher yeast content and makes the body more susceptible to candida symptoms, such as thrush. |
| Brown pasta and brown rice. | Excellent roughage, cleans out the intestines helping to prevent constipation. |

| What's best to eat? | Why? |
|---|---|
| **Seasonings** | |
| Fresh herbs, ginger root, garlic and spices. | All herbs have beneficial, health giving properties. |
| **Dairy** | |
| Small amounts of good quality whole non-homogenised milk and organically produced dairy products such as yoghurt and cheese. Use plain yoghurt and add fresh or dried fruits. | Products made from organically reared animals will not contain the harmful toxins and growth hormones that interfere with our health. However, cow's milk is designed for calves who grow rapidly and is not ideal for humans.<br><br>Adding to plain yoghurt avoids the problem of buying ones full of sugar and additives.<br><br>The fat molecules of homogenised milk are made smaller and pass through the gut wall leading to more allergic responses. |
| Goat's and sheep's milk products are preferable. | These are more easily tolerated than cow's milk products. |

# Here are some useful suggestions:

- At each meal, try to eat something grown in the ground, e.g. potatoes, carrots, onions, sweet potatoes, something grown above the ground, e.g. courgettes, peas, green vegetables, salad, cucumbers, and something from trees e.g. nuts, seeds, fruits.

- Keep a jug of washed celery in the kitchen. You will be surprised how quickly it disappears! Eat a stick while preparing the meal or even afterwards. It has enzymes that help digest your food.

- Keep a bag of organically grown carrots (very important they are organically grown as carrots very readily absorb chemicals in the soil) and have a good peeler so that, in a second, the carrot is cleaned and ready to be eaten raw. Prepare a few at a time and make carrot sticks, keeping them for snacks in a jam jar in the fridge.

- Start every meal with a piece of raw vegetable or fruit as this contains enzymes to help digestion and the immune system. Although cooking food makes it easier for the body to digest, it does trigger an immune response in the body as cooked foods are treated as an invading organism.

- Steaming vegetables preserves the most nutrients.

- The quality of food is more important than the quantity.

When you eat is as important as what you eat. Eating nothing all day followed by a big meal late in the evening is a bad habit. This leads to poor digestion, acidity and excess weight. It is essential to eat breakfast (doesn't have to be immediately on rising). Lunch, ideally, should be the biggest meal and supper should be a light meal eaten at least three hours before going to bed. This gives the body time to digest it properly and provides fuel for optimum functioning. Food eaten late remains undigested for hours providing fuel that is not needed and therefore stored as fat. Chewing well is also important. Food should be chewed to a watery pulp before being swallowed. According to Chinese medicine, we need to chew each mouthful forty times! Try counting yourself. Chances are, you are way off the mark!

Chewing well is also important. Food should be chewed to a watery pulp before being swallowed. According to Chinese medicine, we need to chew each mouthful forty times! Try counting yourself. Chances are, you are way off the mark!

## What water should I drink and how much?

If we know that our bodies are made up of between 60 -75% water (depending on body weight and age) then we realise how important it is to keep up our intake of this vital substance. We start out as babies and children at our highest levels and gradually dehydrate as we age. This is because our thirst mechanism becomes less efficient and we confuse thirst with hunger and eat instead. Dehydration is often the cause of tiredness, headaches and illness, generally. Be aware also that an average glass of tap water can contain many harmful chemicals such as chlorine, fluoride, heavy metals, etc.

Many of you will now be saying, "But, surely, we need chlorine and fluoride." So let's look at what these substances really do. Chlorine is a powerful oxidiser and not only kills micro-organisms, it also oxidises and attacks the DNA in all living matter. This can cause damage that will eventually result in permanent cellular alteration such as aging and cancer. As well as this, chlorine reacts with organic material in our water to produce a family of harmful compounds, which, even in low concentrations, has been directly linked to the long-term development of cancer. Therefore, we don't want it for ourselves and we certainly don't want it for our babies.

Let's turn now to fluoride. The aluminium and phosphate industries produce waste products, one of which is Sodium Fluoride. This is used as the "fluoride" in the water supply, but what is less well known is that it is also used as a rat poison. It is known to be more toxic than lead and only slightly less toxic than arsenic – yet it is being put in our water supply, ostensibly to prevent tooth decay. Most disturbing for our babies is a link between fluoride intoxication and lower IQ levels in children and even chromosomal abnormalities, lowered immunity, thyroid imbalance, heart disease and cancer. And, adding insult to injury, there are no convincing scientific studies to prove that fluoride prevents this tooth decay! Indeed, a recent study by the University of Arizona revealed that "the more fluoride a child drank, the more cavities appeared in the teeth!"

It becomes patently obvious therefore, that the water we drink should be free of all these substances. The contamination and abuse of water supplies generally is one of the main contributions to the "sickness" of our planet. To give one example, an oil used in the electrical industry leaches PCB's (polychlorinated biphenyls) into the sea and water supplies from spillage or breakdown of old electrical appliances. In 1978, PCB's were identified as hazardous to our health and to the environment, but it was not until 1990 that the UK and other North Sea States agreed to phase them out and destroy them by the end of 1999. This became law at the beginning of May 2000. Unfortunately PCB's do not break down and are now in our seas and water supplies. This is just one example of the many contaminants that there are and how long it takes legislation to remove pollutants from being used, how or whether they degrade is another issue. So it is best to drink water that has been filtered through a rock bed formation such as a "wellness water" filter system or use glass bottled mineral water (no plastic bottles!).

In addition to this, I must include the incredible work by a Japanese researcher, Masaru Emoto. In his book "The True Power of Water", he shows through the use of water crystal photographs, how water stores vibrations. He then goes on to show how important it is for us to pay respect to water and believe it or not, he shows that if we say the words "love" and "thanks" each time we use, consume or see water, we will help make this world a better place. Off the wall? Well, take a look for yourself! All I know is that patients who were sceptical about it, have found amazing results. So when you run the tap or pour a glass of water, look at it for a moment and appreciate it saying silently to your self "thank you".

The body needs to replace water that is continually lost through the skin and lungs and other normal bodily functions. I recommend two litres/three and a half pints or more, daily, depending on body weight. This is in addition to water used in beverages such as herbal drinks. It means water, on its own! All other beverages such as tea, coffee, juices and fizzy drinks dehydrate.

Water should be consumed at room temperature. Drink two large glasses on waking, drink another one mid-morning and mid-afternoon and make sure you drink a glass half an hour before each meal. Keep water away from food. Don't make the meals the time to consume your two-litre quota as it dilutes the gastric juices, slowing down and weakening digestion. As your body becomes used to regular water supplies, you will become more aware when you are thirsty.

## What other drinks are beneficial?

Water is best of all. It makes everything work well whether it be our brains or our bowels!

Herbal teas are excellent, especially made from fresh ingredients such as mint, rosemary, or lemon verbena. All herbs have healing properties, enhance our immune systems and help our digestion. Dried herb tea bags are good, although they never equal the fresh herb itself. Tea can be made from fresh root ginger and is very alkalizing and very cleansing. Lemon or lime tea is another beneficial drink and is very refreshing, it helps to break down any mucous in the throat. Mix ginger and lemon together when you have a cold.

Fresh Herb Teas: cut a sprig of rosemary or a small piece of mint, basil, lemon verbena or thyme and place it in a mug or teapot and pour boiling water on to it. Infuse for five minutes.

Ginger tea: There are two ways of making it. Cut and peel a slice, place in a mug and pour boiling water onto it. Or place several slices in a saucepan, cover and bring to a boil, then simmer for five minutes. You can keep the pan and reheat it later on.

Lemon or Lime tea: A slice or two of lemon or lime can be added to water, either hot or cold.

Freshly prepared vegetable and fruit juices can be made with a juice extractor and all sorts of combinations can be mixed together. Carrot, apple and celery are a good combination, or carrot, apple and ginger. Most vegetables work.

# Can I get all the minerals, vitamins and essential fatty acids from my food?

In short, the answer is no. The world's soil has been depleted from centuries of over-farming and intensive use and consequently has been drained of its natural mineral supply. The farming industry attempts to make good with fertilisers, however these contain principally potassium, phosphorus and nitrogen and not all the essential trace minerals. Increased food storage and transportation times, as well as food processing and harvesting unripe produce, have also lowered nutrient content.

A report from a US Senate Document (no. 264) states very clearly that we cannot get all the nutrients from our food. Since then, further research has shown how mineral deficiency in soils causes crop failure. The alarming fact is that foods (fruits, vegetables and grains) now being raised on millions of acres of land that no longer contain enough of certain minerals are starving us, no matter how much we eat. No person today can eat enough fruits and vegetables to supply their system with the minerals required for perfect health, because the stomach just is not big enough!

Physical well being is more directly dependent upon the minerals we take into our systems than upon calories or vitamins or, indeed, the precise proportions of starch, protein, or carbohydrates we consume.

Minerals are essential. They act as catalysts starting the many chemical processes in the body like "the match that starts the fire." They play a crucial role in every body process from circulation to digestion. They also help maintain the acid/alkaline balance of the body. It is critical to our level of health. No bacteria, virus, parasite or fungal infection can live in a healthy, ph balanced body. Excess acid invites them in and they in turn create their own acidic wastes making the host even more imbalanced. Everything we eat, apart from vegetables and fruits, creates acid except for minerals. As the body struggles to alkalize, it will pull minerals from within the system if supplies are not adequate. For example, calcium and magnesium are taken from the bones giving rise to diseases such as osteoporosis later on in life. Deficiencies show up in poor teeth, narrowing of the dental arch, poor growth, poor digestion and muscle development, poor energy, aches and pains, excess weight, as well as a lowered immune system. A minerally deficient, acidic body will never achieve Wellness.

Due to our exposure to pollution and toxins in general, as well as waste from our body's metabolism, we need to supplement our diets with antioxidants. These help soak up the damaging free radicals that attack our cells all the time. There are water soluble and fat-soluble antioxidants. The key ones that are generally written about in the press these days are: vitamins A, C, E, co-enzyme Q10 and the minerals selenium, zinc and fish oils.

The digestive tract houses both beneficial and non-beneficial bacteria. If we have enough of the "good ones" like acidophilus, then these will keep in check the "bad ones" like Candida. Due to the prolific use of antibiotics, to stress, illness and flying, most people need to supplement with a probiotic formulation with all the strains to restore this delicate balance. And looking ahead, a baby's initial supply is entirely due to its mother's levels.

Many scientists now believe everyone needs to increase their intake of nutritional supplements and outlined below is a general guide. Remember, for long term planning for the best health possible, a new baby wants to be born with a healthy stock of minerals. However, minerals may be difficult to absorb, so a liquid supplement of ionic (small particle) minerals that achieves high absorption rates is recommended.

- Liquid mineral and vitamin drink, free from toxic metals;

- Hawaiian Noni juice with active polysaccharide properties;

- Aloe Vera also with active properties;

- An essential fatty acid* formulation that balances the omega 3 and omega 6 oils, needed for every single cell and binds with the toxins stored in the fatty tissues;

- Vitamin C with bioflavonoids;

- Anti-oxidant formulation that includes maritime pine bark, pycnogenols, grape seed extract and combines both the water and fat soluble properties, binds with the toxins and carries them out of the body;

- Vitamin B complex;

- Prebiotics and Probiotics needed to promote the healthy bacteria in our intestines;

\* Essential fatty acids (EFAs) are frequently mentioned in this book. They are SO important. Fish oil contains the performed DHA (dicosapentanoic acid) which is so vital all through our lives but even more so during pregnancy and breastfeeding. The different forms of essential fats can be made from the oils found in nuts, seeds and unrefined, cold pressed oils, but supplementation is necessary. The quality of your baby's skin, the functioning of the brain and immune system are all indicative of how much was given to the baby whilst it was developing.

## What foods and drinks must I avoid?

As a rule of thumb, avoid all processed, refined, adulterated, empty foods and drinks, as well as preservatives, additives, flavourings, colourings, preservatives, bulking agents and carbonated acid drinks. Many of these additives have not been tested in combination with each other and how they affect us is largely unknown. It is a good idea to remind oneself every time we put something into our mouths with this thought: Is this beneficial for me? And how close to nature is it? Here I have grouped together, in tabulated form, some of the key items to avoid.

| What must I avoid and recommended alternatives? | Why? |
|---|---|
| White bread, white pasta, white rice.<br><br>Replace with unrefined versions, wholemeal and brown. | White may look nice, but it is empty and sterile. |
| Fast and fried foods, preservatives and additives. | MSG (Monosodium Glutamate) is used as a flavour enhancer and appetite stimulant, especially in Chinese food. Always ask if it is used and request your food to be prepared without it. |
| Hydrogenated fats<br><br>Change your chocolate to one using cocoa butter, you will be surprised how chocolate addiction disappears when you do this. | These are processed fats heated to very high temperatures; they block the metabolic pathways and absorption of the essential fats.<br><br>Research carried out at Tommy's Maternal and Foetal Research Unit at St Thomas' Hospital in London has revealed that eating a high fat diet when pregnant could lead to unborn baby girls experiencing cardiovascular problems later in life, even if their own diet from birth is balanced and healthy, i.e. when in the womb they may be "programmed" to develop cardiovascular problems. Also, nutritional imbalance in the womb may lead to Type 2 Diabetes in adulthood. |
| White sugar | This is so processed that although it may taste nice, it is volatile fuel giving sudden energy peaks and later leading to dips in blood sugar levels and a low, even depressed, feeling. It is then a vicious circle where the instant solution seems to be eating more of the same without realising that it is in itself the cause of the problem. |

| What must I avoid and recommended alternatives? | Why? |
|---|---|
| Plastics in general and cling film/plastic wrap.<br><br>Don't freeze your plastic water bottles with water or heat food in the microwave using plastic containers or cling film especially with foods that contain fat. | This is because plastics release carcinogenic, highly toxic chemicals called dioxins, which go into the cells of our bodies. Carcinogens cause cancer.<br><br>Dr Edward Fujimoto, manager of the Wellness Programme from Castle Hospital recommends using glass, Corning Ware, or ceramic containers for heating food. You get the same results without the dioxins. If used in an emergency, TV dinners, instant ramen and soups, etc, should be removed from the container before heating. |
| Foods cooked in a microwave. | This way of cooking destroys the nutritional value of food, altering the food's nutrients enough to cause worrying changes such as increased cholesterol levels and white blood cells (immune system activation) in the blood. |
| Aspartame | This sweetener is neurotoxic and breaks down into formaldehyde, a substance used to preserve dead bodies. Cut out all "lite" or "diet" foods that contain any artificial sweeteners. |
| Saccharin | Another sweetener known to cause congenital malformations and cancer in animal studies. |
| Tea, coffee and carbonated drinks. | Caffeine found in tea, chocolate and fizzy drinks dehydrate the body leaching valuable minerals. |
| MSG (monosodium glutamate) | A flavour enhancer that also stimulates appetite. It does this by making bland food tasty, upsetting the controlling (pituitary) gland that leads to obesity and lethargy. Giving MSG to babies may lead to diabetes in adulthood. |

| What must I avoid and recommended alternatives? | Why? |
|---|---|
| Tartozine | A colouring used mainly in soft drinks. Can cause mental and physical problems. It binds with zinc (a mineral vital for healthy growth) and draws it out of the body. |
| Benzoates | Used in soft drinks, beer, salad dressing, jam and causes hyperactivity especially in children. |

To be on the safe side and as a rule of thumb, avoid all food additives: colourings, refined salt, flavour enhancers, preservatives and bulking agents. Many of these additives have not been tested in combination with each other and the effect on the unborn baby is, to a great extent, unknown.

## What about alcohol consumption?

Alcohol, a mild diuretic, forces water out of the cells causing dehydration. It robs the body of essential nutrients, especially vitamins B and C, minerals, magnesium, calcium, zinc, chromium and essential fatty acids. It is also, as everyone knows, an intoxicant. This latter effect occurs when too much is taken in too quickly. The stomach cannot keep pace with the intake, so it is by passed, going straight into the bloodstream and on to the brain and the liver.

The effect in the brain initially causes a feeling of intoxication and euphoria and then, as more alcohol is consumed, motor function, balance and speech control are lost. The liver, often referred to as the body's poison filter, detoxifies the alcohol in the bloodstream. Overload this, or any filter and you get a build-up of toxins with the short-term consequence of headaches, nausea, a general feeling of illness and the longer term consequences of permanent damage to the liver along with the associated damage to the body's system. Later on, fatigue occurs due to the energy reserves being used to deal with the sudden intake. Lastly, sleep itself is disturbed. Quality sleep has several brain wave patterns, but for some reason, alcohol blocks out the REM (rapid eye movement) wave. So sleep is not so refreshing as some might assume.

Alcohol is fattening. Each gram contains seven calories, more than any other kind of food except fat itself and ironically, it stimulates the appetite. Is this why restaurants always serve alcohol?

People can become alcohol dependent because it temporarily relieves some unpleasant symptoms such as depression, tiredness, irritability, tension, inability to think and lack of energy. This is because its sugar content gives a quick burst of energy. However, low blood sugar levels most likely magnify all of the undesirable symptoms in the first place, due to a poor diet essentially high in refined carbohydrates and a lack of water. The short-term relief offered by alcohol only makes the situation worse to the point where food itself is no longer desirable. It is far better to improve the diet and supplement with extra nutrition.

Reduce alcohol consumption on a regular basis: if you drink more than one unit every evening, then start by missing every other night or only on weekends. Go for quality rather than quantity and always have a glass of water first.

Following a wholesome diet, one that stabilises blood sugar levels, will help enormously. A vegetable juice fast can normalise blood sugar levels even faster and can stop the addictive tendencies. To do this, use a juicer to extract all the fluid from vegetables without destroying the health giving enzymes. This speeds up alkalizing the body. Supplement with a multivitamin and mineral formulation, essential fatty acids, a B complex formulation and herbs such as milk thistle and dandelion to cleanse and repair the liver.

# What about smoking?

Smoking is a causative factor in many diseases, reducing not only the length of life, but also the quality, too. The first cigarette is usually very unpleasant. Poisons are introduced into the body resulting in nausea and perhaps a headache. After a few attempts at smoking, however, the body slowly becomes used to the poisons (our survival mechanism) and the addictive effect of nicotine takes hold. Nicotine is a highly addictive drug and once the addiction is established the body continues to demand its fix. Combine the physical biochemistry with the psychological aspects and the habit is thus established.

Considering some of the biochemical aspects, cigarettes affect the circulatory system in several ways. After only one cigarette the heartbeat is increased by 20 – 25 beats per minute. This increases the load on the heart and increases the blood pressure. The heart itself requires more oxygen due to the increased workload, however, at the same time the carbon monoxide from the cigarette forces the oxygen from the bloodstream, depriving the heart of the oxygen it needs. Six hours must lapse before the circulatory system returns to normal. For the smoker who has the last puff just before going to bed and the first puff on waking, this system is normal for only a short two hours out of the entire 24- hour day. This results in respiratory illnesses and even more commonplace illnesses such as colds, sinusitis, bronchitis, emphysema, as well as cardiovascular and circulatory conditions.

Low tar, low nicotine brands are no better. It usually means consuming more cigarettes in order to give the body its adequate fix, as well as ingesting more carbon monoxide and more additives (to give flavour) than regular ones and they do not reduce the risk of heart disease or lung damage.

Smoking aggravates diabetes, ulcers, glaucoma and is a causative factor in osteoporosis, high blood pressure, lung cancer, miscarriages, stillbirths and abnormalities in babies. Taste, smell and vision are all impaired in smokers. This affects their food intake, resulting in less appreciation of natural and subtle tastes and a reliance on heavy seasoning including too much salt to compensate. Skin also ages quicker and a smoker usually has an unhealthy pallor so they go for a suntan to conceal this factor. They need to wear glasses or contact lenses earlier than would otherwise be required. Smoking also produces an insulin reaction that creates low blood sugar, resulting in fatigue, irritability and the desire for another cigarette, setting up a vicious cycle. Smoking destroys the body's supply of vitamin C. Each cigarette will destroy up to 25 mg of vitamin C. Humans can no longer produce vitamin C themselves. It is believed that this is one of the major reasons for much of our ill health and general deterioration as we age. So destroying what precious amounts we take in from our food is very serious.

Now let's look at the psychological aspects of smoking. Associations become ingrained with, for example, having a good time at a party, or the end of the meal, or sharing the habit with a friend or partner added to which smokers rationalise their smoking habit to themselves such as "I like to smoke." What they really mean is they like the "fix" or feeling to which their body has become accustomed. Or they may use the reason "I think better with a cigarette!" This actually is nonsense because smoking constricts the blood flow and oxygen to the brain, making thinking less clear. It is more likely that they are buying time and in meetings or in confrontational instances it shows up as nervousness. Or "A cigarette calms me down!" Again this makes no sense, as after only one cigarette tremours in the fingers increase 39 percent. The insulin response with consequent irritability and fatigue causes adrenal exhaustion and nervousness, not calmness.

The main difficulty with giving up the habit is the lack of success. Many smokers have tried cutting down, unsuccessfully. This route is likely to lead to failure because the body has become accustomed to the addictive substance and it will just make you crave more. Each time the effort to stop fails, the more entrenched the habit becomes which leads to depression and lack of self-respect. A vicious cycle is then set: the habit is programmed not only bio-chemically but also mentally, too. The subconscious will continue to dictate to the person that they need a cigarette unless they address this, too.

The very first step is to decide to give up! Nobody can make someone give up unless they decide to do so themselves. Others can encourage, but the decision has to come from within.

The next step is to seek assistance. Hypnosis and acupuncture are just two of the many therapies that will help. The British Stop Smoking Association, BSSA, has specific programmes such as EasyStop.co.uk. Allen Carr is another very successful programme.

Combine the above with the Wellness Action Plan. A good diet helps maintain constant blood sugar levels, preventing much of the energy fluctuations that stimulate the desire to smoke. A high level of vegetables, raw carrots, vitamin and mineral supplementation, as well as increasing the water intake, speeds up the removal of the toxins and alkalizes the body. Vegetable juice fasting can speed up the withdrawal process.

Cut out coffee (often a cup of coffee and a cigarette go together) and do not just substitute sugar or sweets instead of smoking. It increases the chances of failure.

## Are there harmful ingredients in our everyday products that I need know about?

Every year up to 400 million tons of chemicals are produced and a thousand new substances are created. Individually, each chemical used in a minute quantity may be harmless, but there is growing concern about their combined effects. They accumulate in our fat cells, another one of our protective mechanisms as these substances can do less harm in our fatty deposits than in our organs. What is crucial to remember in this context is that when pregnant these fat deposits are mobilised to provide fuel for the growing baby. As a consequence, some of these unwanted chemicals are reintroduced into the mother's blood stream and so into the baby's blood stream. What's more, we don't even know what some of these chemicals can do. We are dealing with a minefield.

How to check for harmful ingredients:

Have you ever considered that you are poisoning yourself just by washing your hair and cleaning your teeth? Did you know that whatever products you put on your face are absorbed into your skin? That's only the beginning of it. Go through everything you use. Start with the bathroom. Anything that has sodium lauryl sulphate, sodium laureth sulphate, propylene glycol, talc and aluminium must go. Check every item from toothpaste to mouthwash (alcohol must be avoided) to shampoo, conditioner, deodorant, face creams, make-up and nail varnish and even sun creams.

Here are some commonly used ingredients to be avoided in the personal care industry:

- **Alcohol:** a colourless, volatile liquid, which can cause body tissues to be more vulnerable to carcinogens. Mouthwashes with an alcohol content of 25% or more have been implicated in mouth, tongue and throat cancers.

- **Alpha Hydroxy Acid:** used to exfoliate the skin and, in the process, damages skin cells and the skin's protective barrier.

- **Aluminium:** a metallic element used widely in antiperspirants, antacids, antiseptics, aspirin, lipstick and cosmetics. Aluminium toxicity affects the bones, kidneys, stomach and brain. Research links aluminium to Alzheimer's disease, Parkinson's disease, dementia and even breast cancer.

- **Animal Fat (tallow):** used extensively in bars of soap, acts as a breeding ground for bacteria.

- **Artificial Musks:** found in cosmetics and perfumes and have been linked to cancer.

- **Bentonite:** porous clay that expands to many times its dry volume as it absorbs water. It is used in many cosmetic foundations that can clog the pores and suffocate the skin.

- **Collagen:** an insoluble fibrous protein that is too large to penetrate the skin. The collagen found in most skin care products is derived from animal skins and ground up chicken feet. This forms a layer of film that may suffocate the skin.

- **Dioxins:** a group of toxic chlorinated chemicals formed as a by-product from many industrial processes including bleaching paper. Dioxin treated containers sometimes transfer dioxins to the product itself. Dioxin is "the most potent carcinogen ever studied" according to K. Erickson. Exposure during pregnancy can cause birth defects. These hormone disruptors can be found in many personal care products such as feminine hygiene products: tampons and sanitary towels, shampoos, creams, deodorants and antibacterial soaps, often as a result of leaching from the plastic containers.

- **Fluorocarbons:** a colourless, non-flammable gas or liquid that can produce mild upper respiratory tract irritation. Fluorocarbons are used as a propellant in hairsprays.

- **Formaldehyde:** a toxic, colourless gas that is an irritant and a carcinogen. When combined with water, formaldehyde is used as a disinfectant, fixative, or preservative. Formaldehyde is found in many cosmetic products and conventional nail care systems.

- **Fragrances:** Many different ingredients are used, far too many for labelling purposes and are often synthetic and derived from petroleum products. Some are very dangerous such as Toluene, a neurotoxin and glycol esters linked with infertility and birth defects.

- **Glycerine:** a syrupy liquid that is chemically produced by combining water and fat. Glycerine is used as a solvent and plasticiser. Unless the humidity of air is over 65%, glycerine draws moisture from the lower layers of the skin and holds it on the surface, which dries the skin from the inside out.

- **Kaolin:** fine white clay used in making porcelain. It smothers and weakens the skin.

- **Lanolin:** A fatty substance extracted from wool and used in many cosmetics and toiletries. Often causes allergic reactions and skin rashes.

- **Lead:** found in hair dyes, cosmetics and contaminated water. Lead toxicity leads to damage in the nervous system, kidneys, bones, heart and blood and poses greatest risk to infants, young children and pregnant women as it affects growth.

- **Lye:** Used to make bars of soap. It corrodes and dries out the skin.

- **Mineral Oil:** Derived from crude oil and is used industrially as a lubricant. On the skin, it suffocates the pores and therefore prevents the skin from breathing and eliminating. This ages the skin and dries it out even more.

- **Propylene Glycol:** This is a mineral oil used in brake and hydraulic fluid and antifreeze. It glides over the skin easily making it appear to be moisturising. However, it is a humectant. This means it retains the moisture content of the skin, again suffocating the skin and stopping it from breathing and eliminating. Material Safety Data sheets warn users to avoid skin contact with propylene glycol as this strong skin irritant can cause liver abnormalities and kidney damage.

- **Phthalates:** found in fragrances, make-up, shampoo, nail polish, soaps, even baby toiletries and is a powerful endocrine disruptor. According to Dr Samuel Epstein from the Cancer Prevention Coalition there is evidence that phthalates induce birth defects, low sperm counts and other reproductive toxicity in experimental animal studies. There is a link between phthalates and early puberty in girls where they show early signs of puberty before eight years of age: breast development or pubic hair and in boys, abnormal genital growth.

- **Sodium Lauryl Sulphate (SLS):** This is a harsh detergent used in industrial floor cleaners and engine degreasers. It is known to be a skin irritant and is rapidly absorbed and retained in the eyes, brain, heart and liver, which can result in harmful long-term effects. SLS could retard healing, cause cataracts in adults and prevent children's eyes from developing properly.

- **Sodium Laureth Sulphate (SLES):** This is the alcohol form of SLS. It is slightly less irritating but may be more drying. Both SLS and SLES may cause potentially carcinogenic formations of nitrites and dioxins to form in shampoos and cleansers by reacting with other ingredients. Large amounts of nitrates may enter the blood system from just one shampooing.

- **Talc:** A soft grey-green mineral used in some personal hygiene and cosmetic products. Inhaling talc is harmful as this substance is recognised as a potential carcinogen. Its molecular formula is very similar to asbestos.

- **Triclosan:** a hormone disruptor with possible liver damaging effects and is found in toothpastes, deodorants and antibacterial soaps.

**Make-up.** What chemicals are in your cosmetics? Check from the list above and avoid using anything you are not sure about. You may find lead (a heavy metal known to cause abnormalities in developing babies) in lipsticks, talc, eye shadows and blushers as well as many of the toxic ingredients listed above in many of the well-known cosmetic brands. Here is a test you can do yourself:

1. Put some lipstick on your hand,

2. Use a gold ring to scratch on the lipstick;

3. If the lipstick colour changes to black then you know the lipstick contains lead;

4. Change where you shop! (See resources).

**Household cleaning products** are also loaded with harmful ingredients. Some of the combinations are quite lethal and are known to cause burning fumes to the delicate tissues of the lungs. Avoid aerosols. These contain chemicals that can actually damage the nasal membranes. Air-fresheners and aerosols can even cause diarrhoea and earache in babies and children and depression in mothers. Laundry detergents and fabric conditioners are also another arena full of toxins. Do not use harsh, biological formulations and avoid fabric conditioners/softeners. Residues from detergents and softeners stay in our clothing and bedding, contributing to abnormal skin conditions. Children who suffer from asthma have improved dramatically when their bedding was washed without softeners as their body heat releases harmful fumes from the resulting impregnated chemicals.

In addition, there are also some very dangerous chemicals in our homes, which come from flame-retardants and plastics. Look out for and avoid where possible:

- **Polybrominated diphenyl ethers:** used on furniture, clothing and TVs.

- **Perfluorinated compounds:** found in non-stick pans and water-resistant clothing.

- **Oestrogen mimics/Hormone Disruptors:** found in plastics, cling film, bottle tops, tin cans, water pipes, plant pesticides as well as those already listed. Dr Margret Schlumpf, an environmental toxicologist, recently assessed sun creams and found that of the ten tested, nine contained oestrogen mimics. The advice to pregnant and lactating women is to not use them.

Change your shopping habits and find cleaning and personal care products that are free from these harmful ingredients. Some companies will deliver directly to your home. Throw out non-stick pans and avoid using plastics as much as possible in the kitchen, especially cling-film or cling wrap.

# What are geopathic stress and electro-magnetic pollution?

Science shows quite clearly that the earth emits energy waves that are harmful to humans. It is known as Geopathic Stress and is caused by the earth's radiation from natural rock formation, fault lines, underground streams and excavation holes and cavities. We can't see, hear, or touch these waves, so it does not occur to the vast majority of people that the land on which their home or work place is built could be harming them. These wavelengths interfere with our cell-to-cell communication system affecting our health and are linked to a number of symptoms including cancers, autoimmune diseases, joint pains, short-term memory loss, panic attacks, nightmares, insomnia, migraines and headaches, irritable bowel syndrome, thrush, hormonal imbalances, cot deaths and infertility. Geopathic Stress is widely recognised in parts of Europe whom even have areas tested by state-registered dowsers (people who use rods or pendulums to help locate these harmful wavelengths), but it is largely ignored in the UK.

Then there is Electro-Magnetic Pollution, man-made pollution that comes from electricity and electrical products. The following appliances all cause this pollution: electric blankets, electric radio/alarm clocks, coiled spring mattresses, answer machines, transformers, halogen lights, hairdryers, microwaves, fridges, music centres, computers, wall plugs, mobile phones and power lines, pylons and mobile phone masts. Sometimes the combinations of the above can cause electromagnetic stress that disturbs the pineal gland in the base of the brain. This affects sleep patterns and the body's ability to regenerate as well as the hormonal system.

What is most alarming is that the place where we spend approximately a third of our lives, our beds, could be most at risk from both Geopathic Stress and Electromagnetic Pollution. As we step into our cosy beds in anticipation of waking refreshed, our bodies may be battling away with a constant barrage of disturbing energy fields, preventing regeneration, repair and proper body functioning. Imagine that your cells are trying to talk to each other, but louder and bigger voices drown their voices. What an exhausting time. No wonder we don't feel well when we wake!

# *So what's to be done?*

Have your home checked for Geopathic Stress.

Consider your use of electrical appliances around the home, removing any unnecessary ones where possible, for example, the radio/alarm clock. I always recommend removing the microwave oven altogether as it changes the molecular structure of the food with disastrous consequences. Never microwave milk, especially not formula milk. Make sure all electrical appliances in the bedroom are switched off at night at the mains with the wall plugs pulled out. When using a lap top computer, run it off the battery not the mains – less electro-pollution - and always shut down at night. Do not leave any appliance on standby. By reducing electro-magnetic pollution, there is the added benefit of cutting down on energy consumption, thereby reducing carbon emissions that are harmful to our environment. With regard to mobile/cell phones, there are devices that reduce the negative frequencies. When dialling from a mobile, hold the phone away from your ear while it is ringing and use the loudspeaker until they have answered.

Electrical appliances to switch off at the wall socket when sleeping:

1. Electric blankets

2. Radio/alarm clocks

3. Telephones, answer phones, rechargeable and portable phones

4. Computers, TV and music centres

5. Avoid microwave ovens altogether

6. Mobile phones or pagers (do not keep switched on all the time)

## Case History

Cindy, 37, had suffered from extreme exhaustion and was diagnosed as having Chronic Fatigue Syndrome, five years ago. She had become so bad that she could barely walk, going upstairs had become impossible and she could no longer live any sort of normal life. She moved in with her parents who had moved to a bungalow, knowing that this would be easier for her. Cindy lived on state benefit and the generosity of her parents. She had had enough and was desperate. To try and come to me for a consultation was impossible and even talking on the telephone brought her out in a sweat. So I put her in touch with an eminent dowser, a scientist who belonged to the British Society of Dowsers. He discovered that she had an underground water stream running below her bed, her coiled spring mattress was giving out high electro-magnetic waves and she had every type of electrical gadget in her room. The very same night, she moved her bed and slept on a futon, removed as many electrical appliances as possible and unplugged the rest from the wall. The next day, she had slightly more energy but it took six weeks for her to notice a significant difference. She then was able to visit me in the practice and started on the wellness programme and now she is a completely different woman. What's more, she has become an apprentice dowser and she aims to further her studies so that she can help others.

## What about day light and electric light?

We need approximately 30 minutes of sunlight daily without sunglasses, glasses, or contact lenses so that the light cannot just reach the skin (2% absorption) but the retina too (98% absorption). The small amount that enters our skin is vital because the body develops vitamin D, essential to calcium absorption for our bones and teeth. By obtaining enough light our bodies function at optimum levels and we reduce the associated risks such as depression, tiredness and more serious illnesses such as immune disorders and cancer.

Electric lighting can be very damaging to our health, especially ordinary fluorescent lighting. Studies in schools have shown that under this type of lighting, students demonstrated fatigue, hyperactivity, irritability and lack f concentration. Whereas other students exposed to full spectrum lighting fter replacing the fluorescent tubes in identical controlled conditions vere calmer with much improved academic achievement. Furthermore, hildren with learning disabilities overcame their reading and learning roblems. Another surprising phenomenon is those children who were xposed to full spectrum lighting developed two thirds less dental cavities han the children in the room with the ordinary fluorescent lighting. Ordinary yellow/orange lighting emits a frequency that makes us crave arbohydrates, feel depressed and irritable, effects menstrual cycles and he immune system. Is this why we crave munchies in the evenings?

Aim to be outdoors as much as possible with an absolute minimum f 30 minutes daily, ideally in sunlight. Literally grab every opportunity. Allow the light to enter the eyes directly, so remove sunglasses, glasses and ontact lenses.

Did you know that we have junk lighting? Most lighting emits redominately a yellow/orange, flickering light which upsets our energy alance and is detrimental to our health, whereas full spectrum, flicker-free ight contains all seven colours of the rainbow in a balanced spectrum. So ill your home and work environment with quality light. Buy full spectrum, iigh frequency light bulbs, now also available as energy saving.

Do not use ordinary fluorescent lights. If they are in the work place, hen suggest that alterations be made. Incidentally, the rays from TVs hit he retina, interfering with the brain wave patterns that promote healing. Listening to the TV does not affect the brain in the same way, so if you are ll, don't sit in front of the TV.

## *Do your teeth affect your health?*

Yes. It has been known in conventional medical circles that bacteria n the mouth can go into the blood stream and cause illnesses. One in articular is streptococcus haemolyticus, which can cause inflammation in he heart itself. So never neglect your mouth. Teeth are made up of living lusters of tiny crystals, which actually absorb energy from the food before t even reaches the stomach. The blood flows into the centre of each tooth through the nerve and tiny bundles in the dentine. For teeth to remain healthy, it is not just about good oral hygiene but excellent nutrition with plenty of minerals.

By eating empty, hollow foods that taste nice but have no nutrient value, we force our teeth to part with their minerals for more urgent use in other areas of the body so they become weaker. Add bacteria and plaque build up and watch the rot set in.

Some dentists know the state of a person's health just by looking inside their mouth. Each tooth represents different parts of the body. So when there is a problem in any tooth, the corresponding part of the body will be affected.

Putting metal into the mouth is not the best solution. In some people, this can create a sensitivity or an allergy and if it is very bad, this can lead to immune disorders such as chronic fatigue, muscular aches and pains, chronic and unexplained conditions.

## What type of exercise should I do? And how do I make time for it?

Exercise helps to give a good supply of oxygen, which is the ignition factor in burning energy from the foods we eat. A good supply is always necessary for the healthy functioning of the body's metabolic pathways. When we have a good supply, we feel well and vibrant, think clearly and have plenty of energy. If we do not receive enough, we feel depressed, tired and generally unwell and unfit.

Today, there is less physical effort in our everyday lives than there was a century or so ago, due to all the technology and machinery at our disposal. We have washing machines, cars, vacuum cleaners and such, all of which have reduced our physical exercise and exertion on a daily basis. Yet the body was designed for movement, so we need to work out ways to do so.

We need to stretch and realign ourselves weekly through regimes such as yoga, Pilates and Alexander technique. These systems help unravel the areas of tension and blockages that prevent blood flow and keep the spine and joints supple.

We also need a rhythmical and sustained form of exercise known as aerobic exercise that increases our heart rate and our lung capacity as well as our immunity to disease, such as swimming, brisk walking, Nordic walking, cycling, hiking, rowing and running. Thirty minutes of such aerobic exercise five times a week boosts the production of our immune defending white blood cells.

I advise people to find simple ways of exercising within their daily lives such as running up the stairs instead of taking the lift or walking round the block in the lunch break or after work. Exercising does not mean we have to spend masses of time in the gym, it is far better to walk for 30 minutes in the fresh air, which gives us the added benefit of daylight rays. This prevents us from becoming depressed due to lack of daylight.

## Are you currently at your ideal weight?

Here, we have to be honest with ourselves, even though there are tables and guide lines, each one of us knows whether we are carrying extra weight or not. Excess weight is becoming more and more of a universal problem. This is due to a number of factors including our lifestyle. Our lives are more sedentary, we live on convenience fast foods which are devoid of essential vitamins, minerals and essential fats, we eat too much, too often and in a hurried, stressful manner, stretching the stomach wall so that the receptor cells are unable to send efficient signals back to the brain and we often eat late at night. We eat when we are tired, often before we sleep and yet it is far better to go to bed on an empty stomach. Additionally and importantly, we don't drink enough water between meals.

What we put in our mouths must be digested. Any chemicals that cannot be broken down go to the liver. As the liver becomes overloaded, it dumps these into the cellular matrix and into our cells, a home for chemicals and non-food substances housed away from the vital organs. As this process continues, accumulation increases, the body starts to function less well, we become more acidic, then add dehydration, lack of nutrients, lack of exercise and life style factors and more and more fat builds up. No matter how much the individual reduces their intake, weight never seems to go, or the weight comes back as soon as it is lost.

This is where the understanding of how our thinking affects our results comes into play. The body and mind are programmed to maintain balance. Look at our blood temperature for example. As soon as the outside temperature changes, then either more blood or less blood will flow to our extremities. So it is with our minds. Subconsciously, the body is conditioned to be a certain weight. If this is not addressed when the weight changes, then no matter how much or how little we eat, the cells will automatically take us back to where we were in the first place, which may not be the desired result. As a result, so many people just give up and accept being the wrong weight.

The first step is to decide to do something about it and then find a photograph of yourself when you were slim. Pin it up on your mirror so that you look at it every morning and evening. Close your eyes and hold this picture in your mind and imagine how you would feel if you were that same weight now and able to wear clothes in your ideal size. Cultivate this feeling so that every time you feel overweight, you counter this negative one with your ideal positive one. It helps to write down your goal, in the present tense and by when you want to achieve it. Literally date it. All this helps to programme a new image of you in the subconscious mind.

Now, by applying the principles of a wholesome diet with supplements, by eating and chewing food in a relaxed manner, by drinking enough water and exercising ideally before 11 am (helps put the body into a fat burning mode), you have a greater chance to lose the weight. Follow the detoxification guidelines using the detox kit to speed up the process. When your body is free of excess acids and toxins, it has no reason to hold onto the extra weight, providing you believe you can!

# *How do you see yourself?*

We need to ask ourselves some personal questions. What are our attitudes and beliefs? Are you an optimist or a pessimist? Do you anticipate disaster or success? Are you a dreamer or realist? Do people warm to you or do they shy away? Are you a good listener? Do you ask a question with genuine interest or just out of politeness? Do people relate to you, confide in you and respect you? Do you believe you are capable of setting out what you intend to achieve? Do you support yourself? Do you encourage yourself? Do you pull yourself down and say, "Well I never thought it would work anyway?" It is by observing what we say to ourselves, our continual internal chatter, that we can raise our awareness and cultivate new belief systems to make choices that will cultivate Wellness.

Everyone holds a mental picture of himself or herself. Whether we are aware of it or not is a different story. Examining how we think is just a start. We then need to delve deeper into the subconscious mind and find out what picture you have stored of yourself. You have to put a plan together mentally first, before any physical change can occur. It is no good saying, "I'm going to drink more water," and then do nothing about it. After first deciding what to do, we then have to visualize ourselves in our minds doing it and programme our subconscious mind with this new picture. Then it will be a question of doing this every day until a new habit is formed. We are creatures of habit, therefore, it necessary to reprogram ourselves with good ones.

To alter your subconscious mental image, you need to:

1. Build a picture in your mind of how you want to be, create a portrait of yourself. For example: a person who makes the necessary changes in life style to achieve Wellness, a person with a positive state of mind, someone who set targets and achieves them, someone who has self-respect and integrity, someone who has loving relationships and so on.

2. You then take this a step further and make a written portrait of yourself - how you want to be. Stick this up on your mirror and every morning and evening, read it out aloud. The written word will then imprint itself on your subconscious mind (memory box) and will actually help you attract into your life what you are aiming to achieve. This process is very empowering as it fosters self-belief. Often, the challenge in making changes in life can be put down to not having self-belief.

Some people try to alter their results by their actions alone and the truth is you can't. We need to change our thoughts and mental image as well. As our actions are governed by our subconscious mind, in order to change our results we need to change the picture we hold in our minds.

## What negative feelings should I avoid?

Negative feelings arise from negative thinking. Such thinking triggers a subconscious memory and in a nano second, the emotion ripples through our energy field and body chemistry causing toxic pollution. Be aware of the following negative emotions:

- **Fear:** This arises when we are unable to cope or when we feel inadequate. The best thing to do is to face the fear and ask yourself, "How would I deal with it if it happened." Having faced the fear in your mind the powerful emotion then dissolves. Fear creates tension in the body, especially the kidneys and lower back.

- **Hatred:** Hatred breeds hatred. Stay away from whatever or whomever you hate, as this negates it.

- **Jealousy:** Usually means that, in your own eyes, you are inadequate and unworthy of affection.

- **Greed:** Whether for food, power, or affection, it usually comes from a fear that you are not capable or worthy of obtaining these for yourself. You have to be a giver not a taker.

- **Envy:** Emotional pain that arises from another person's success. Sometimes you simply ask yourself the question: Would you want their troubles and trials too? Usually the answer is no and then you can move on to determine what prevents you from obtaining the things you envy. Usually, it is due to fear of failure.

- **Resentment:** Suppressed anger, which eats into the body and can lead to cancer.

- **Possessiveness or superiority:** It is utterly evil to possess a person. Let go!

- **Guilt:** Usually manifests as pain, as if you are guilty you are expecting punishment and pain is the body's way of giving punishment.

- **Criticism:** Someone who is continually critical needs to relax and let other people be.

All these things stem from fear of one's own inadequacies. This is muddled thinking. Everyone has unique gifts and talents; it is up to us to find them and decide how to use them. If we are constantly comparing ourselves to others, then we will never be happy. Happiness has to come from within. Listen to your inner voice. Listen to your heart where only understanding and love exists. The story goes that we have two hearts, a black one and a gold one and according to which one you feed will be the one that dominates your life. Negative emotion and negative thinking feeds the black one and positive emotion and positive thinking feeds the gold one. So let's decide to feed and nurture the gold within.

Be aware of these negative feelings; they cause ill health and misery. Notice when they creep into your life and if they do, work with yourself or a professional to help you understand why you are experiencing them so that they can be resolved. By acknowledging them, it is then possible to let them go and any ill health that has been caused as a result.

This does not mean you should never experience any negative emotions. It just means you have a better understanding of how to deal with them. For example, if you are angry you can count to ten and calm yourself down so that you do not add fuel to the flame. Be aware of the damage you can do when you are emotionally out of control. In fact, anger usually arises in situations when something is out of your control.

## How do I stop worrying?

Worry is a deadly force. Why? Because it is a waste of time and it often spirals out of control. Recognise that worry has a negative effect on your life. It robs you of your strength and if you catch yourself saying you "can't do it" quickly, flip the switch in your mind to "I can do it." Ninety two percent of the things we worry about never actually happen anyway, so don't waste your energy. When you find yourself worrying, pull yourself up sharply and concentrate on a mental activity, build a positive picture, feel it and expect it to happen. Stop worrying by changing the routine in the mental gym. Instead, build a wonderful picture of the desired result.

*"A person cannot directly choose his circumstances,*
*but he can choose his thoughts and so indirectly,*
*yet surely, shape his circumstances."*

**James Allen 1864-1912**
Author of *As a Man Thinketh*

## Explain what detoxing is all about. What do you recommend?

The body detoxifies every second. It is something that every single one of our hundred trillion cells does, whether we are aware of it or not. However, the level of efficiency of our cellular detoxification is directly related to our level of health. Wellness IS about improving this level so detoxifying, or helping, the body to remove waste and toxins is an integral part of this approach. This is why it is so important to be aware of what we put into ourselves either via anything ingested or by products we use on our skin or absorb from our environment. Everything that has been discussed in this step aims to help the body function efficiently including the removal of wastes and toxins.

To understand this further, let's take a look at the two main sources of toxins:

Waste produced in the body as a by-product of metabolism, the process of cells absorbing nutrients and excreting wastes.

Toxic material absorbed in food, drink, heavy metal poisoning and through the lungs and skin, pollutants from the outside world.

These toxins have to be removed from the body via one of the following main exit routes: the bowel, the kidneys and urinary tract and the lungs. If these become sluggish or blocked then the rubbish flows over into the other eliminative channels: the skin, the mucous membranes, menstrual blood, the lymphatic system and the liver. When this happens, our immunity decreases and illness and disease occur. Here are just some of the early symptoms of toxin build up: skin problems, anything from rashes, spots to psoriasis, menstrual cramps, pain and discharge, swollen glands, over acidity, excess weight, lack of energy and tiredness, indigestion, constipation, headaches, food cravings, addictions, blood sugar imbalances, hormonal imbalances, cellulite, difficulty sleeping, allergies, pain of any sort, depression and moodiness. If this internal muck is not cleared out, we literally rot away and it is no wonder that the strain on the tissues and organs leads to chronic illness such as cardiovascular disease, arthritis, cancer, immune disorders, digestive and organ disintegration and ME.

So we need to spend time and energy not only keeping ourselves clean and well groomed on the outside but also clean on the inside. A word of caution here: we need to prepare the bodily exit routes first before pulling the toxins out of the tissues and organs. Otherwise they can simply flow round the system and back into the tissues again.

Start by drinking 1.5 litres/2.5 pints of still water every day to flush out the urinary tract. Improve your diet by cutting out the obvious rubbish such as take-away food, white flour, sugar, coffee, fried food and alcohol (just for a while!). Take a brisk 10 -20 minute walk outside in the fresh air every day (helps not only with blood circulation but with the lymphatic system also). Deep breathing and standing up straight also helps not only the respiratory system but the lymphatic system, too. Encourage sweating either from exercise or a sauna as this helps eliminate metabolic wastes and toxins through the sweat glands.

I recommend a modern homeopathic detox kit for one or two months, depending on how much toxicity there is in the body and then a three day fruit fast followed by a parasitic detox (see website: www.viviencleregreen.com/detox).

Lymphomyosot - aids in draining lymphatic system,

Berberis Homocord – aids in cleansing urinary tract,

Nux Vomica Homocord – aids in cleansing digestive tract.

Use 10 drops of each 3 times daily in a large glass of water.

## *Three Day Fruit Cleanse*

Choose a three-day break and fast for three days on organically grown apples or grapes. Drink as much water as you like, but a minimum of 3 litres/5 pints. Chew each mouthful well. Do not do any strenuous exercise but have a daily walk outside. Get early nights and enjoy a good book rather than sitting in front of the TV or computer. It is ideal to have a massage at this time. If you have never done a cleanse before, start with one day and then repeat it a week later. It is not nearly as difficult as it sounds!

After this you should be feeling much cleaner, lighter and more clear-headed. It is recommended to do a detox once or twice a year.

There are many holistic treatments and therapies. The most important point is that you find something that you like and a therapist/practitioner that you trust who is coming from their heart, so to speak. Avoid any healing that has off-the-body work. Always insist on hands-on-the-body work. Below are listed some of the treatments that I recommend:

**Acupuncture**: Acupuncture is a system of healing which has been practised in China and other Eastern countries for thousands of years. It is used to treat people with a wide range of illnesses by balancing the energy levels round the body. This is done by using very fine acupuncture needles, which when inserted cause a tingling or a dull ache, but not pain. It is, in fact, a very effective way of removing pain from the body. The principle aim is to balance the whole person and not just treat the symptoms.

**Aromatherapy:** Massage with essential oils is an ancient healing art. It is a relaxing and revitalizing treatment, stimulating blood and lymphatic flow, as well as combating aches and pains and fluid retention.

**Hypnotherapy:** Helps to relax the state of your body.

**Flower Remedies:** They can help emotional blockages. Australian Bush Essence She Oak, in particular, is good for improving ovulation and pregnancy.

**Herbal Medicine:** Herbs are prescribed to help the body to heal, repair, detoxify and remineralize. The overall effect is to restore the body functions to optimum levels.

**Reflexology:** A science based on the principle of energy zones and reflex areas in the feet, which correspond to different parts of the body. The reflexologist works by applying thumb pressure to specific points on the feet which unblocks congested areas, regulates body organs and systems, stimulates circulation and lymphatic drainage and generally restores balance.

**Metamorphic technique (a spin-off from reflexology):** stimulates the spinal reflexes along the outer ridge of the feet and the hands. The practitioner can trigger energetic changes that include ridding the body's cells of their memories of past traumas and disturbances to remove emotional and physical blocks. Quantum physicists have now proven that there is a vibrating energy field that connects us all, known as a morphic field. Mothers who have this treatment throughout pregnancy generally have an easier birth with very calm babies.

**Nutrition:** Profiles are made of the individual to assess what levels of nutrients they are deficient in and what they need to be healthy and as efficient as possible.

**Homotoxicology:** Complex or modern homeopathic preparations (known as antihomotoxic medications) are used to treat out genetic inherited toxins, amoeba, fungal infections, parasites, viruses and bacteria and to stimulate and balance the functions of the body. Usually a biofeedback machine is used to test the different points on the hands and feet to identify the cause of any imbalance. For example, Chlamydia Trachomatis is a bacterium that in 70% of women and 50% of men produces no symptoms. Yet, this can be a cause of infertility or miscarriages. It can be picked up and eliminated.

**Homeopathy:** is an exceptionally safe form of naturopathic medicine, which treats the whole individual. It is equally concerned with maintaining good health as well as aiding recovery from ill health. Like all forms of medicine, even those which use powerful drugs and high technology surgery, homeopathy relies on the body's own powers of self-regulation and self-healing.

Most people, when they are ill, suffer not only from the basic diagnostic symptoms of the disease but also from other symptoms, which are specific to each person. In orthodox medicine, these individual symptoms are mostly unimportant. But in homeopathy, they are vital for giving the correct prescription. In fact, there are over 3,000 homeopathic remedies to-date. This is why different patients may receive different remedies for the same disease.

**Osteopathy:** restores the musculoskeletal system of the body to a state of balance and harmony. When there are problems in the framework of the body, not only are there aches and pains in the joints and muscles but blockages prevent optimal functioning of the other systems including the internal organs. Correction releases these blockages.

**Paediatric Osteopathy:** (as defined by the Osteopathic Centre for Children) is based on the principle that all ailments - whether minor or serious - are as a result of an imbalance somewhere in the network of the body's systems. A paediatric osteopath will use manual techniques to bring about profound changes within the child's body through gentle manipulation.

This will allow the different body systems - the nervous system, the immune system, the muscular system and the circulatory system - to work effectively and optimally. The treatment uses no drugs, and is non-invasive.

**Cranial Osteopathy:** is a very gentle form of treatment, which involves feeling the rhythmical cycle of the body fluids and energy fields. The skull is made up of 26 bones which are joined in such a way that allows this rhythmical cycle to be felt and can be adjusted by a trained practitioner.

# *Conclusion*

The challenge in today's society is how to sift out and deal with the flood of information and advice on so much such as what to wear, what to drink, or what to eat. If we go back to when I became interested in this field, the popular press was low fat, low protein and plenty of carbohydrates. Now twenty-five years later, we are told that carbohydrates are the least essential part of our diet and we should keep them to a minimum. In between have been countless other fads: little and often versus two meals a day, no dairy, no meat, eat fish and now be careful it is polluted. Press and papers continually flood us with snippets, offering up different foods or even the same foods as either causing or preventing cancer or heart disease. There are endless diets for losing weight and over the years we have been lead to believe that to lose weight we must avoid fat. Now we are told to eat fat to keep thin. How do we steer ourselves through this maze of conflicting advice? I believe it comes back to working in harmony with nature and then to balance sensitivity and awareness of our unique, individual needs.

This is why Wellness is really a voyage of self-discovery. We learn to discover how we operate both physically and mentally. It's all about finding out what suits us, looking for signs of imbalance early on and of wrong or muddled thinking caught up with negative emotion. As Oscar Wilde says, "To love oneself is the beginning of a life-long romance."

## Two Families

Now to illustrate Wellness in a practical way, let's take a look at two families who came to the practice for advice on health matters for their one-year-old babies. June, a young woman of 29, brought Mark to see me. She wanted a general check-up. Mark was a healthy looking baby with beautiful soft, silky skin, an even coloured complexion and sparkling eyes. He sat contentedly on his mother's knees throughout the consultation, playing with the car key and her watch. June told me that he slept well at night and had a good morning sleep and occasionally dozed off in the car. He was crawling well now. She had weaned him slowly on to purees of fruits and vegetables and didn't introduce wheat until he had his first back molar tooth. He had, however, picked up a stomach bug two weeks ago and had been quite ill for two days and then rather listless for another couple of days. He had recovered well. June wanted to know whether he needed any supplements such as vitamins and minerals and whether she was giving him all he needed. She had breastfed him very successfully after having a few difficulties at the beginning and now she just fed him at night before he went to sleep.

Now let's look at another baby of the same age, a boy called Gary. He was a fat, pale-looking baby who seemed rather miserable and very restless. Marian, aged 33, his mother was very distressed by his skin condition. He had eczema over most of his body. At night, she had to wrap his arms and legs in bandages to stop him scratching and causing his skin to bleed. He did not sleep well and both his parents had become very exhausted. She had tried the usual creams and medications from the doctor but was concerned that if she kept using the cortisone cream that it could have long-term effects. (I personally have seen several adult patients whose skin had been damaged in this way). Marian did not know about introducing foods slowly and had put him on most foods by the time he was seven months. Gary also appeared to suffer from constipation and was not able to crawl but just shuffled on his bottom. Marian felt there must be something that she could do to help her young son.

These two babies show a marked difference in their health and I always ask for information about the parents' health and whether they did any pre-pregnancy preparation.

June, the mother of the first baby had come for a consultation BEFORE she became pregnant. She wanted a general check-up. In doing her profile, I learned that she suffered from constipation, headaches and period pains, but otherwise she was in good health. She usually skipped breakfast and grabbed a sandwich in her coffee break at work, or she would wait till lunch when she usually had a salad and vegetable soup. She and her husband cooked supper with freshly prepared ingredients. They did not eat processed or ready prepared meals. I explained that constipation meant toxins and waste were building up in her intestines causing putrefaction and acidity and that she must sort this out before becoming pregnant. The headache and period pains could be linked to her constipation due to waste matter sitting in her intestines. So I advised her to drink two litres/three and a half pints of purified water daily and to start her day with a cup of boiling water with a slice of lemon and ginger. Also important would be to eat breakfast, this helps to stimulate the peristaltic waves for bowel movement. She could eat some fruit with either some live, whole yoghurt or porridge and banana. I also prescribed a general vitamin and mineral supplement, an antioxidant and essential fatty acids. When her constipation had ceased, I talked about a cleansing diet and a six-month programme before trying for a baby. June was quite happy to carry out this advice.

Her husband, John, 33, was an Insurance Adviser and led a fairly stressful life and loved sports. He played football for his county when he was younger and was involved in coaching children at his local club. So he knew about the importance of being fit and well. He agreed to June's suggestion of coming for a general check-up before they conceived.

The results of John's health profile showed that he did not sleep well and he had problems with his knee due to an old football injury. He skipped breakfast and lived on endless cups of tea throughout the day. I explained that prolonged stress would disrupt the proper functioning of his body as it would be constantly sending out messages to slow or shut down systems that are not necessary in the immediate moment of survival. For example, digestion is inhibited, repair and healing slows down and blood pressure goes up together with blood sugar and energy imbalances; the body will be constantly on the alert for the "enemy," hence disturbed sleep.

John and Jane followed the pre-pregnancy programme for the recommended six months making the necessary changes to their diets like eating breakfast and drinking two litres/three and a half pints of water daily. They both went through a detox program and made decisions to change some of their shopping habits to remove harmful chemicals and formulations from the home. They also took the nutritional supplements I recommended.

I received a call from June, seven months later to tell me that she was pregnant! She had conceived the first month they had tried. Now she wanted to know if I would guide her through the next stages of pregnancy and birth. I explained that this was very much part of the whole process and that it would be a pleasure.

June went on to have a relatively straightforward pregnancy with a slight hiccough when blood tests showed that she was anaemic and that she should take iron supplements. We reviewed her mineral supplementation and decided she needed a liquid tonic rather than iron tablets, which can be very constipating and not necessary. So once this was sorted, she continued with her yoga classes and read up about childbirth to find out what her options were. In the end, she decided to go with the birth unit attached to her local hospital. She found that there were a great team of midwives and although she was apprehensive, she was informed. So when John rang to tell me that she had delivered a beautiful, baby boy weighing 7.12 lbs naturally, without any medical intervention, I was not surprised but thrilled for them all.

Now let's take a look at the other baby's parents' histories.

Marian was overweight, had aches and pains in her joints and suffered from hay fever, constipation and PMT (pre-menstrual tension). She was also bothered that her skin still erupted in outbreaks of spots and blemishes, after all she was 33. Her diet consisted of very little fruits and vegetables and no fish at all. She found that she was so tired that she had little energy for cooking so they lived on processed foods and sometimes could not overcome her cravings for chocolate. She liked swimming but found it was too time consuming now that she had a baby.

Her partner, Kevin, was an electrician. He was also overweight, with huge fluctuations in energy levels. Sometimes he almost fell asleep in the car when he was driving and he kept a permanent supply of chocolate and sweets in the car to keep himself awake. He worked long hours and, sometimes, found his job very stressful. He would often pick up a take-away on the way home from work.

Marian explained that she had terrible problems getting pregnant. There was no explanation for her infertility so she had gone for IVF (invitro fertilization). It had failed twice, but finally on their third attempt, it worked. And to their joy, they now had Gary. She had felt terrible during most of her pregnancy, very sick at the beginning and had put on even more weight. As for the birth, she did not go into labour on her due date and so when she was offered the option of being induced, she readily agreed. She did not know that it would speed up and intensify the contractions, which made it more painful, so she had an epidural in an emergency situation. The baby was delivered with forceps, as she was unable to be in an upright position and use gravity to help her. She had tried to breastfeed but did not establish it well at the beginning. And once she had introduced formula milk, the baby lost interest in feeding from her.

When I explained that many of the causes of these problems were caused from the lifestyle choices she made, namely her diet and mineral, vitamin and essential fatty acid deficiencies, she was shocked. She had no idea that she could have prevented many of her problems and that her skin outbreaks and constipation were linked and was even more horrified to learn that had she known she could well have prevented her son's current distress. He was clearly deficient in essential fats and minerals for a start and his body would be contending with the empty, hollow food he was currently eating. I also explained that excess weight could raise oestrogen levels and prevent ovulation (oestrogen is one of the hormones that carries a message to the pituitary gland which affects the release of the egg stimulating hormone). The aches and pains she felt in her joints were partly from the excess weight she carried but also be due to allergies caused by a leaky gut. This is when the digestive system has become inflamed or damaged and allows toxins to get through into the blood stream. A self-help way of checking the most common allergens of wheat and dairy is to avoid them completely in the diet for two weeks and then introduce a lot of dairy at one meal and watch for symptoms. Continue avoiding both again and then a few days later to repeat only this time overloading on wheat. Many allergies can be overcome once they are eliminated for at least four months together with protocols for healing the body. It is usually advisable to seek professional help for this.

The best reassurance I could give her is to let her know that the body is programmed to regenerate and heal, it is amazing how quickly it can. So we set out an action plan for dietary and lifestyle choices. To begin would be a bit strange, but once a commitment is made these new choices can become tomorrow's habits. Both she and Kevin agreed to drink two litres/3 and a half pints of water daily, to start off with a healthy breakfast (dietary advice), to gradually increase their fruit and vegetable intake and to cut out refined, processed and fast food as much as possible. We added a liquid cocktail containing vitamin and minerals, as well as Hawaiian Noni juice.

As far as the baby, Gary, was concerned, the following advice was given: change his formula milk to a goat's formula (nanny's goat milk infant formula) as the fat molecules of goat's milk are closer in size to human milk than cow's milk; to introduce freshly prepared and pureed vegetables into the lunch and tea time meals; to use soft, ripe fruit at breakfast and as a mid morning snack; to supplement Gary's diet with a fish oil supplement and liquid minerals; to remove all chemicals such as sodium lauryl sulphate, propylene glycol, mineral oils, petroleum derived chemicals and talc from the bathroom products and to change over to washing powder that did not leave chemicals in the material that could irritate the skin or release vapours from his body heat into his lungs. I also suggested treating the skin topically with almond oil.

It took a few weeks, but eventually Gary's skin healed so well that you would not have known he had a skin problem. Marian also noticed that Gary's behaviour completely changed. He was calmer, he slept through the night, cried far less; and he was crawling (very important for good brain development and physical coordination). Marian and Kevin gradually improved themselves too and to her astonishment, she lost weight following the Wellness Diet although it is not aimed specifically for this. I explained that once the body is fed properly, weight imbalances would not only normalise but stabilise too.

These two stories illustrate how two families with baby boys of the same age journeyed into parenthood, one with knowledge in advance and one without this benefit. Just look at the end results. Both resulted in a huge difference, not only in their own health but in their children's too. This book is devoted to making sure you, the reader, have this journey explained well enough in advance to avoid some of the pitfalls and needless suffering caused by such lack of knowledge and understanding. This book is devoted to helping you to make informed choices through all the various stages.

*"For prevention to be effective, it needs to be targeted at the point when it can make the most difference"*.

**Sue Gerhardt**
Author of *Why Love Matters*

# Step 2 - Pre-Pregnancy

Preparation for pregnancy lays the foundation of Wellness for both the mother-to-be and the as yet unconceived child. It is absolutely essential that both parents, but especially the mother, are in good health before starting on this journey. Did you know that how a mother gives birth and welcomes the new born lays down the foundations of its emotional well being for the rest of it's life? Did you know that most malformations are caused from the male side? Did you know that most ovarian and testicular cancers can be traced back to the toxicity of the mother's womb? Did you know that overcrowded and narrow mouths are caused from mineral deficiencies from the mother and the father? Did you know that digestive disturbances and heart and circulatory disorders have their beginnings in the mother's womb? Did you know that IQ levels could be increased through supplementing the mother's diet both before and during pregnancy?

Step 2 is what needs to be done in addition to the Wellness Action Plan before conception by both the prospective mother and father to ensure the best for the babies as yet unconceived.

# How long should a pre-pregnancy programme be?

A six-month programme is recommended, longer if possible. This is the time to look ahead and plan the journey into Motherhood, to create a poison-free womb by detoxifying and preparing the body and mind before conception for both the future mother AND father. As it takes two to make a baby, it is vital that the future father is also aware of his own health and plans to eliminate toxins. After all, his sperm contributes to half the embryo! It helps hugely if he understands some of the mental/emotional issues involved with pregnancy, such as the importance of keeping his partner happy and calm for the future well being of his baby. What to eat and drink and other guidelines for a healthy lifestyle, covered in the Wellness Action Plan of step 1, are not repeated here, but the reader does need to use this information in addition to the following advice and recommendations.

# I know it sounds vain, but what will happen to my figure after I have had a baby?

Most mothers-to-be voice this concern privately to themselves, it is a natural concern. A woman's body has the ability to adapt and expand to carry a baby and to give birth. Providing a woman takes care of herself and follows a healthy lifestyle according to the Wellness Action Plan guidelines, then there is absolutely no reason why a woman should not regain her figure. The usual concerns that are voiced to me in the practice are: "It will ruin my boobs", "My stomach will never be flat again", "I have seen other women's bodies after they've had babies and they look terrible", "I don't want stretch marks" or "I have heard your cellulite can get worse." The truth is that you reap what you sow. If you have neglected yourself, eaten an empty diet devoid of vitamins and minerals and not taken care of yourself during pregnancy, then these things can occur.

# Will having a baby spoil my sex life?

Most definitely no! On the contrary many women say it becomes even better! Sometimes there are misconceptions about such things that need to be aired. Over and over again in this book you will read that a woman's body is designed to have a baby and if you work in harmony with nature then all will be well. One of the amazing things about natural childbirth is the vagina stretches and becomes more elastic so the baby can pass through the birth canal, but afterwards it tightens up back to normal. However if there has been surgical intervention and cutting, then there is a risk of scar tissue forming and a certain loss of sensation.

# Do you suggest a cleansing/detoxing diet before conception?

Yes, most definitely. We all have in our bodies between 300 and 500 synthetic industrial chemicals that would not have been there 50 years ago because they did not even exist! Most of them collect and accumulate over the years in our fatty tissues, sometimes for our entire lives. The problem is that they are mobilised in pregnancy and can be passed onto the next generation via the mother's blood flow through the organ that feeds and nourishes the baby, the placenta, thus creating a toxic womb.

These harmful ingredients interfere with the baby's growth and development. Studies now show that serious diseases such as breast and testicular cancers can even be traced back to the mother's womb. However, not all is doom and gloom. We can do something to prevent this by cleaning up our internal and external environments, by removing the harmful chemicals, by taking in good nutrition and excellent supplementation before, during and after pregnancy and by following a cleansing/detoxing diet before conception. Women who have followed this plan avoid many unpleasant symptoms including sickness. But to cleanse/detox during pregnancy must not be done as there is a high risk of moving these toxins from the stored fat cells and tissues into the mother's blood stream and hence to the baby.

We need to stimulate and activate the eliminative channels. We are talking about the bowels, the kidneys and urinary system, the lungs, the skin (the largest eliminative organ, sometimes known as the third kidney), the lymph system (responsible for removing the waste products from our cells) and the liver which all need cleaning out on a regular basis.

In the practice, I recommend a detox kit for one or two months depending on how much toxicity there is in the body, followed by a three day fruit fast and finally a parasitic detox. The kit consists of:

**Lymphomyosot** - aids in draining lymphatic system,

**Berberis Homocord** – aids in cleansing urinary tract,

**Nux Vomica Homocord** – aids in cleansing digestive tract.

## *Three Day Fruit Fast*

For three days, eat only organically grown apples or grapes and chew each mouthful well. Drink as much water as you like, a minimum of 3 litres/5 pints. Do not do any strenuous exercise but have a daily walk outside, get early nights and enjoy a good book rather than sitting in front of the TV or computer. It is ideal to book a massage treatment during this time.

If you find the three days too much of a challenge, start with one day and then, a few days later, do it again. It is not nearly as difficult as it sounds!

## *Parasitic Detox*

There are various bowel cleansing formulations on the market but only some of these include anti- parasitic preparations (see website).

# *Are there any tests that can assess my state of health?*

In the practice I use tests to assess people's levels of health, mainly from the following four.

• Hair analysis,

• Root hair analysis,

• Homocysteine testing, or

• Metal testing, for example Melisa,

These tests give a very good indication of your general state of health and I recommend a visit to your local holistic practitioner who will know how to identify which of the tests you need.

The pre-conceptual charity, Foresight, uses hair cut close to the root for mineral analysis, as hair root analysis captures the very signature of the person. To check your homocysteine levels, a simple blood test can be done from home and sent off to a lab or by your doctor. A healthy body will produce low levels of this damaging toxin, a by-product of eating protein and should really be broken down further into beneficial nutrients. This biochemical process can only occur if there is enough B2, B6, B12, folic acid, zinc and magnesium. If those vitamins and minerals are minimal, then high levels of homocysteine will result. It is vital that this is not the case during pregnancy to ensure a really, healthy baby.

It is far easier to clear any metal toxicity before pregnancy. Metal toxicity has the potential to cause autism. If this toxicity is not cleared out of the mother's body before pregnancy, then the toxicity will have to be cleared out of the child's body later on which can be problematic.

# *I understand that I need to avoid harmful ingredients, but is there anything further I should consider at this stage?*

This is covered fully in the Wellness Action Plan, but as part of the pre-pregnancy programme we have to be more careful at this time, so I recommend the following in addition to removing harmful chemicals from our homes and workplaces:

**At the Hairdresser:** Take your own hair products with you so as to avoid any harmful ingredients going into your blood system and ultimately into your baby's. Ideally, keep your hair as natural as possible avoiding hair dyes, bleach and perms unless using safer plant-based alternatives. Maintaining a good cut will make you feel good in the meantime.

**Beauty Treatments:** It is vital that you are aware of chemicals that are used in the majority of these treatments. Stick to aromatherapy that uses good quality, unrefined carrier oils, such as almond, jojoba and coconut and essential oils that have healing effects, suitable for pregnancy. The following oils are not suitable: cedar wood, chamomile, clary sage, ginger, jasmine, juniper and rosemary.

**Manicures and pedicures:** Believe it or not, whatever you put on your finger and toe nails ends up in your bloodstream. The nail breathes and this will be blocked by most proprietary nail polishes and treatments, including the application of artificial nails! Best of all is to leave nails in their natural state. For special occasions, use breathable varnishes and safer artificial gel nails.

# Should I give up alcohol before becoming pregnant?

Yes. Both you and your partner need to avoid alcohol completely for four months before conception. It will make a huge difference in the quality of the man's sperm and make the woman's womb more fertile.

Alcohol reduces the absorption levels of nutrients and depletes the body of previously stored ones. To give your baby the best start, you and your partner want to ensure the best quality egg and sperm. Alcohol goes straight into the liver (the body's poison filter) from the bloodstream and excess alcohol creates acetaldehyde (a poisonous substance similar to formaldehyde used for preserving bodies). It also reduces absorption levels of minerals and vitamins, especially zinc and B6 which are vital ingredients for cell growth, as well as depleting the body of folic acid, a key nutrient in preventing neural tube defects such as spina bifida. Alcohol affects sperm motility, sperm quantity and quality. It causes impotence and difficulty in achieving orgasm. In men, it can upset testosterone, increasing the level of female hormones. It can also cause chromosomal abnormalities. Babies born to alcoholic fathers can have any number of problems ranging from heart defects, to physical abnormalities (such as webbed fingers), to learning and behavioural problems.

For the woman, alcohol upsets the hormonal balance preventing her body from producing enough progesterone early in the pregnancy and so miscarriage occurs.

Studies have shown that just one drink a day can reduce IQ levels, not only in your child but for the next generation as well.

## Case History

A young single mother, Janice, brought her son Jimmy, aged two, to see me. The first things that I noticed were his face, lips and nose. His top lip was very thin with a strange flattening above it and the bridge of his nose was almost non-existent. He had very small eyes, a squint and large, protruding ears. He was tiny and underweight for his age. Before I even started taking his case history, he rushed at the wall and started banging his head against it several times and then sat on the floor in a rocking motion. He was clearly showing abnormal behaviour.

Janice told me that he was born with Foetal Alcohol Syndrome (FAS). His father, now no longer involved, was an alcoholic and she confessed that Jimmy had been conceived in a drunken stupour. Thus, it was an unexpected pregnancy and she had no idea that alcohol could cause such harm, so much so that she had continued to drink throughout her pregnancy. So it was a shock to find out that both she and the father were the cause of all Jimmy's problems.

Jimmy was a small, premature baby and had to be hospitalised for several months. The bonding process had been interrupted. When he failed to thrive, further tests were carried to reveal a hole in his heart. It was touch and go as to whether he would live or not. Gradually he grew stronger and was able to undergo heart surgery. I also learned that his mouth had not formed properly and that he had a cleft palate. His fingers were joined together in a web like a duck's foot and he had had surgery to help correct this, too.

As a baby, he screamed and screamed and threw tantrum after tantrum. Janice had nearly given up and put him in the hands of the authorities. But in stepped her Aunt Mary who gave her incredible help. As it turned out, this Aunt had come with Janice for her consultation and was waiting in the car in case she was needed. Suddenly, Jimmy started rushing at the wall again, banging his head and knocking over nearby objects. It was impossible to continue the consultation with him in this state, so Janice took Jimmy out to the car so we could continue.

So we started at the beginning of the Wellness Action Plan and outlined suggestions and ways to improve this little boy's health and well-being. First of all, his diet and liquid intake needed improving and we took a hair sample for a mineral analysis and tested for the most suitable vitamins, minerals and essential fatty acids. We then addressed the toxins in the bathroom and home environment. I also advised her to see a Paediatric Osteopath at the OCC (Osteopathic Centre for Children in London). Janice was determined to do whatever she could to improve her son's life and we worked together for a number of years. Many improvements took place, but the physical abnormalities could not be undone.

All the above physical and mental symptoms were directly caused by the alcohol consumption of both parents. In fact, sometimes the abnormalities can occur from just an alcoholic father. Further more his early arrival, interruption of the bonding process following his birth and his mother's physical and emotional state contributed to his volatile emotional behaviour.

As a result of the experience Janice has been through, she helps to promote information on FAS so that future parents do not unknowingly damage their children's lives. Had she known what she knows now, she would never allowed alcohol to ruin the health of her child for his entire life.

## *How long do I need to stop smoking before being pregnant?*

Six months. This gives your body time to clean up and get back into balance. Refer back to smoking in the previous chapter for contacts and help.

Smoking is bad at all times but especially at this stage in life as it depletes the body of vital nutrients needed to form a healthy baby such as zinc, selenium and vitamin C. It also introduces lead, cadmium, cyanamid, carbon monoxide, ammonia and thousands of other toxic compounds into the body.

Furthermore sperm is reduced and there is an increased risk of babies born with malformations, hearing defects, abnormal limbs and even leukaemia and cancer in the future child. Researchers at Oslo University even suggest that cigarette smoke interferes with the development of the spine.

Difficulties conceiving by smokers are common. The sperm find it more difficult to penetrate the female egg and swimming to the egg is harder due to the thicker consistency of the woman's mucous.

In summary, smoking leads to abnormal cell replication causing physical malformations such as cleft palate, hare lip, deafness, squints, heart defects, poor growth rate, lowered immunity, bladder and kidney problems, skin and bone disorders, respiratory infections, as well as affecting a child's intelligence and general behaviour. It also increases the chance of cot death. Furthermore it has a knock on effect to the next generation through the genes.

## *I know hard drugs are damaging, but what about grass?*

Avoid it totally. Consumption of marijuana is linked to stillbirths and malformations, impaired mental functioning, reduced IQ, hyperactivity and reduced sperm count.

Where a baby's mother or father uses recreational drugs of any kind, the baby will be born with a very toxic load in its body and huge nutritional deficiencies, which may result in major problems.

## Case History

Ann brought her daughter Amelia, aged five, for a consultation. She was concerned about the difficulties she was having with her. This bright little girl was underweight and very small for her age, but the main concern was her hyperactivity. She was never still for a moment and often showed very violent behaviour and, when upset, she screamed the house down. Diet was also challenging as she was very allergic and if she was given any foods which contained artificial colourings, preservatives or additives it made her even more hyperactive. She never went to sleep easily and often woke in the night and was up and about at 5 am every single day. Her mother, Ann, was exhausted and wanted to know if there was something that she could do to ease the situation.

To understand the cause of this little girl's problems, we needed to know what happened to her in the womb, in other words, during her mother's pregnancy.

It transpired that Ann was not Amelia's birth mother. She had not been able to have her own children; she and her husband had adopted Amelia when she was seven months old. Her birth mother had been a heroine addict and had given the baby up for adoption at birth. The baby was born as an addict and spent three months in hospital while her tiny body overcame this addiction.

There had been no welcoming, loving and secure reception from her mother when she was born, no maternal bonding, no hormonal flood in the "Critical Hour" after birth of the love hormone, oxytocin. No heart to heart feelings of falling in love with each other. Added to which she had had a number of different nurses looking after her in the hospital, preventing a substitute mother bonding/attachment relationship being established. Then she had been fostered until she was adopted by Ann and Peter.

They had all sorts of physical and emotional challenges including feeding problems and food intolerances. Life had been very difficult, to put it mildly, as Amelia could not be taken out easily without screaming and shouting or vomiting up food she could not tolerate. However, she had settled in with her adopted parents very well, but now Amelia was labelled dyslexic, dyspraxic and hyperactive. She was having one-to-one support at her local primary school and she was given a simple diet with no processed or junk foods and wheat, dairy and sugar free. This was another concern because it made socialising very difficult. I explained that with time we could clear out much of the toxicity caused by heroine from Amelia's body so that her system could heal, but it would involve a considerable amount of detoxing through herbs, homotoxicology, diet and the removal of any external toxins.

Ann knew she had taken on a challenge when she adopted Amelia and was determined to overcome the bad start her daughter had been given.

## How long should I be off the pill, contraceptive injections, or implants before I conceive?

Come off the pill and any hormonal contraception for a minimum of six months, ideally for one to two years. Nutritional supplementation is needed to correct the imbalance caused by this chemical hormone. It is important to make sure your hormones are well balanced before conception. Factors which cause further disruptions come from synthetic oestrogen mimics; they are bio-chemically similar to the female hormone, oestrogen. These chemicals are everywhere from pesticides, industrial chemicals, PCB's in electrical products to plastics. So it is vital to remove as much as you possibly can from your home. (See Wellness Action Plan) A book I highly recommend is *Oestrogen: The Killer in Our Midst*, by Chris Woollams.

There are a number of alternative contraceptive methods, barriers, such as condoms and diaphragms and natural family planning methods where you learn to identify when you release the egg (ovulate) so that you can work out your "fertile" days, (usually five days before ovulating and two days afterwards.) There are also predictor kits using urine dipsticks to identify when you ovulate, which are very reliable. There are two key indicators that can be used to help identify ovulation: body temperature and consistency of mucus. For body temperature: buy a fertility thermometer and take your temperature as soon as you wake up every morning. Your temperature will be slightly lower before ovulation then it will rise and stay at the higher level for the next two weeks, falling again as your period starts. The other reliable indicator is your vaginal mucus. Around ovulation the mucus becomes thinner, clearer, more abundant and slippery (looks like raw egg white) as this encourages the sperm to swim through it towards the ripening egg. After ovulation the mucus becomes thicker and cloudy.

The pill depletes your body of essential nutrients such as B vitamins, including folic acid (needed to prevent spinal malformations), vitamin C, magnesium and vitamin A levels. It also increases copper levels which block out zinc, a mineral needed for growth. A number of women using these forms of contraceptive devices take much longer than six months to regulate their systems due to some of the possible side effects such as weight gain, depression and skin eruptions. All this needs to be resolved before conceiving.

## *Can over-the-counter or prescribed medication affect my unborn child?*

Yes and, if necessary, seek the advice of a Nutritionist, Holistic Practitioner or Naturopath. Ask your GP about the safety of any medication and how you can come off it.

The ideal is to be in the best possible health so that you don't need any medication. Some medications actually interfere with ovulation and sperm production preventing fertility. There is a higher risk of chromosomal abnormalities in a developing baby if medication is taken in the three weeks prior to conception.

Most people are aware of the thalidomide disaster but are unaware that many drugs pass through the mother's placenta to the unborn child. The drugs hold toxic substances which should be avoided. Research has shown that aspirin, taken in the first half of pregnancy, has an adverse effect on the child's mental performance, such as lowering IQ levels. Paracetamol also has been linked to cell mutations. Tranquillisers can disturb the brain and nervous system in the early stages of pregnancy causing malformations, mental disorders and brain damage. Anti-depressants also have increased risks to the developing baby. Some drugs interfere with the hormones that stimulate the development of the follicle so that progesterone and oestrogen production is insufficient and leads to a 'blighted ovum' and miscarriage.

Tranquillisers, if used in pregnancy, prevent the neuro-transmitters from working properly so a child is born with lower levels of "happy hormones" and is more likely to turn to addictive substances to raise them later on in life. You don't want to give birth to a natural born junkie!

Recent research (American Journal of Obstetrics and Gynaecology) examined the usage of prescription drugs among a group of 152,531 pregnant women between 1996 and 2000 and discovered that 64% were prescribed some medication and, of these, 40% received a drug for which human safety during pregnancy had not been established. Even worse was that 5% were prescribed a drug that was known to possibly cause some foetal risk.

Use of roactane, a medication used to suppress acne, can cause birth defects.

## What about geopathic stress?

Geopathic stress and electro-magnetic pollution are covered in the Wellness Action Plan but I wanted to share the following story with you because it illustrates very clearly this unseen form of pollution.

Molly had been trying desperately for a baby for a number of years, had twelve miscarriages and had never been able to find the cause. She had, after the first two, looked to holistic medicine for suggestions and recommendations to help the problem and still continued to have miscarriage after miscarriage. Her husband never felt refreshed after a night's sleep and just accepted this as the norm for the past eight years. She eventually called in an advisor to her home to test for geopathic stress and electro-magnetic pollution. She learned that her spring mattress was emitting energy waves unhealthy for humans and there was a magnetic field that crossed her bed in two positions: one was at the point where her uterus was positioned and the other was at her head by the pineal gland. This magnetic field had the capacity to alter messages in her body so that she could not carry a baby and was the cause of all her miscarriages. The bed was repositioned and the electrical devices were removed. Together with extra vitamin and mineral supplementation her body balanced and a few months later she was heavily pregnant and went on to give birth to a very healthy and robust young boy.

## *I remember reading something about dental health in the Wellness Action Plan step one, but could you expand specifically?*

Each tooth represents a different part of the body. Decay in a particular tooth will correspond with a problem elsewhere, so it's important not to ignore signs from the mouth! Decay is not only about poor dental hygiene and food and drink coming into direct contact with the teeth, but it is also about mineral deficiency and energy blockages. Dentists advise brushing and flossing teeth twice daily. It is very important to use a toothpaste and mouthwash, but find a holistic dental care system that is free of toxic chemicals such as sodium lauryl sulphate.

Another concern is silver (amalgam) fillings that can contain up to 50% mercury, described as possibly the second most deadly toxin on earth. Mercury can leak from the mother's fillings into her blood stream and tissues and can cause miscarriage or infertility problems or into the developing baby, causing learning, behavioural, growth and a host of other challenges.

Before you conceive have your teeth checked out by a dentist, but one who is aware of these potential problems. You can have a blood test done which will test for metal sensitivities or allergies. With due care, amalgam fillings can be replaced so long as precautions are taken to mop up any toxic metals released in the process with nutritional supplements such as Chlorella. Go to an amalgam free dentist.

# *Is it important to strengthen my back before being pregnant?*

A woman's body goes through incredible physical changes during pregnancy. So now is the time to get you and your back into shape! Posture is very important and the tendency when pregnant is to arch the lower back and push the tummy out causing great strain on the back muscles. What, in fact, needs to happen when the time comes is to lengthen the spine and tuck in the tummy and baby! This is where the right type of exercise, such as Pilates and Yoga, is so important, In addition it is advisable to see an Osteopath or Cranial Osteopath for a general check-up, thus uncovering any areas that are locked or stressed. Areas to look at are the head, neck and jaw-joint (known as the TMJ joint), lower back, hips and pelvis. Being pregnant means your body has to adjust to make space for a growing baby and the more relaxed and free your muscles are the easier it will be.

Make an appointment with a recommended Cranial Osteopath/Osteopath for a check-up. It may be decided that some other treatment is also necessary such as massage, acupuncture or reflexology.

Another very useful system for strengthening the back is the Alexander Technique. This is an ideal method of re-educating the muscles and helps us to become aware of how we go about our daily activities such as sitting, standing or walking – releasing tension from bad postural habits makes us taller, freer and more elastic and, encourages the baby when the time comes, to be in a good position for birth. Women who have had sessions during pregnancy often have easier births.

Look up the Alexander Technique register to locate a nearby teacher for a session and then decide whether it is something that will help you to continue through your pregnancy. Personally speaking, I know it made a huge difference to me, enabling me to have my babies so much more easily.

# *Is it important NOW to consider the type of exercise that would be helpful in pregnancy?*

Experience shows that women who do the right type of exercise before and during pregnancy are more in touch with their bodies resulting in healthier pregnancies, easier births and recover their figures more quickly. In addition to having stronger more flexible bodies, they are better able to cope with any problems that arise. The best forms of exercise during pregnancy are Pilates, Yoga and Swimming.

Pilates is a form of exercise that helps align the spine and physical structure of the body by strengthening and lengthening the muscles without adding bulk but toning your whole body. It teaches the individual to use the tummy, back and pelvic floor muscles correctly. This is known as core stability. It is a wonderful way to develop a strong back and gives you a great figure. However, you cannot start Pilates in the first three months of pregnancy. The ideal is to start a year before becoming pregnant.

The word "Yoga" means union of the mind, body and spirit. It is based on ancient Indian philosophy of balance in movement, thought, lifestyle and diet. Regular practice of the physical exercises improves posture, circulation, energy, flexibility and strength. Women respond extremely well to yoga in pregnancy and they have a unique and greater sense of body awareness known as propriosensitivity. I highly recommend finding a registered "birthlight" teacher.

Swimming is wonderful exercise when pregnant, especially towards the end as you grow bigger and carry more weight around. The relief of floating has helped many pregnant women for generations! It is not necessary to start before pregnancy unless you are unable to swim.

Daily fresh air and natural daylight makes a difference to our health and an absolute minimum of ten minutes each day is fundamental, take off any glasses and remove contact lenses so that the natural day light rays can enter the eye itself. Even in the middle of the city, there are always green areas. It might mean taking a walk round the block in cold, wet weather, but you will feel better afterwards.

The body burns fat better with exercise earlier in the day. If you are overweight, exercising before 11 am will help put the body into a fat burning mode, even a brisk walk around the block or up a hill or flight of stairs is good - anything that raises the heartbeat for twenty minutes and increases deeper and more frequent breathing.

Take up Yoga or Pilates, or try both and see which you prefer. Find a studio or class in a suitable location and make it part of your regular routine.

It is important to understand that it can be dangerous to over exert oneself in pregnancy and if you are currently doing very strenuous and demanding physical exercise it would be a good idea to wind this down to a minimum and find a more suitable substitute as discussed above.

## *Tell me about the power of thought with regard to pre-pregnancy?*

As explained in Step 1, we become what we think about. In other words, the constant silent talk that goes on in our heads every single moment of the day determines our results. I have advised women to write down this talk especially in relation to becoming pregnant or being a mother. It is extremely revealing.

I know of many people, although physically healthy with no abnormalities, who are unable to become pregnant. It was not until we started looking at what they were thinking and feeling that we found the cause of the difficulty to be coming from the mind. At that point, we were able to take the necessary steps that, fortunately, resulted in successful pregnancies. Here is an example:

## Case History

Maria, 23, had miscarried twice and now was even having difficulty conceiving. She wanted to see if she could find the cause from a holistic point of view. She was a healthy, young woman and, through questioning her, she admitted to being frightened of not being a good enough mother and she was afraid of the future. Her infertility was caused by her emotional fears, which were reinforced daily by her negative thinking and internal chatter. So we worked out a plan to weed out the doubt in her mind and to program her subconscious mind daily by writing out the following meditation twice daily:

*"I give love and thanks for the process of life,*

*I trust and believe in my ability to be a mother.*

*I trust and believe in being able to have a baby.*

*I ask for courage, strength and power,*

*so that I may journey into motherhood with joy and ecstasy."*

We had two further sessions to uncover some of her fears and discover from where they had originated. It actually went back to her own birth. Subsequently she and her mother went out for lunch to discuss this with a very therapeutic result. Later on in the year, when she was on holiday, she became pregnant. She continued to see me throughout her pregnancy and asked me to be her "doula" (attendant) at the birth. She felt that having me there would make her feel more confident to go ahead with a natural birth. Often this is the role of a Grandmother or Mother, but in her case, her grandmother had died and her mother did not feel it was appropriate to be there. I visited Maria just before the baby was due and the moment she felt something unusual she called me. I left immediately. By the time the Midwives arrived, her labour was well established and she gave birth very easily in her own home. It was a very special moment for us all and I felt privileged to be involved.

As discussed at length, mental fitness is as important as physical fitness. Now you might be wondering how this affects your baby's future well being. The body is like a laboratory, continually making chemicals including emotional ones. So when we become angry, a chemical message is sent round the body affecting the cells, which in turn affect organs all linked to that emotion. For example, anger goes to the liver and gall bladder, fear to the kidneys and bladder. The same applies when we are happy and it is important to know this so that your body floods the developing baby with good messages.

## *Are you happy with your life?*

This may sound like a very big question. It is more important than ever to put your own house in order, so to speak, before inviting a new being to share it with you! So, in understanding that our emotions are passed on to our baby, one of the steps is to look carefully at your life before being pregnant. Your circumstances can have a directly negative effect on you. If you allow this to happen say, for example, you are in a job you don't enjoy and you cannot change it, then choose to change your attitude and perspective towards it and find an approach that does give you satisfaction. Make a positive decision to stop blaming and moaning.

Mind mapping is one way to actually see your thoughts and beliefs written out on paper. On a piece of A4 paper turned landscape, draw a circle in the centre containing the words "your life." Now, around the paper, in smaller circles linked to the centre, note the different aspects of your life, your home, your work, your job, your hobbies, your interests, your family and your friends. Next to these smaller circles, write anything related that comes to mind. For example, by home you may write paint bedroom or new kitchen and gradually you will build a picture of many of the aspects of your life.

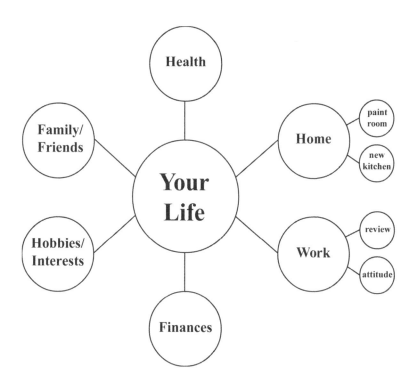

Having done this, examine each area and make an action plan to do something about the areas with which you are not happy. Equally, enjoy the fact that in some areas things are going very well! If you do need to decorate parts of your home, do it before your pregnancy as there can be toxic chemicals released from building materials.

There is a very simple way of approaching problems in life, first to acknowledge them and then how to resolve them. If something can be changed physically, then do it or if not, change your attitude towards it. Remember if you don't do something about the negativity, tomorrow will be exactly the same as today. You and ONLY YOU are responsible for the way you feel.

# *I am having difficulty conceiving. What suggestions do you have?*

So many cases of infertility problems can be overcome by seeking and rectifying the root cause of the problem whether it be biochemical, energetic or psychological. This way much misery and heartache can be avoided. Reasons for difficulties may include:

- Poor nutrition and lack of nutrients, essential fatty acids, minerals and vitamins and/or heavy metal toxicity. Alcohol, tobacco, caffeine (tea, chocolate and cola drinks as well as coffee) decrease the chances of conception. (See Step 1 – Wellness Action Plan);

- Being underweight or overweight decreases fertility. Fertility expert, Harvard Professor Rose Frisch claims: "Many women who maintain the body shape made popular on the catwalks throughout the world are completely infertile." But don't use this as an excuse to become fat. This in itself causes hormonal imbalance, toxic retention in fat cells both causing miscarriage and infertility;

- Geopathic stress and electro-magnetic pollution;

- Stress and attitude to life's situations and circumstances interferes with the hormonal balance necessary for conception. Being aware that your reactions are key to reducing such stress. For example, traffic jams, bad days and failure easily brings out the negative side, but if we are aware that we can choose our reactions to situations, then we can look for something positive. This reduces stress levels enormously;

- Allergies, yeast overgrowth, leaky gut/inflamed or damaged gut lining and parasites;

- Genito-urinary infections are frequently undiagnosed. If there is a bacterial infection in the fallopian tubes such as Chlamydia Trachomatis, it can cause inflammation, which prevents conception or causes miscarriage.

- Polycystic ovaries are a common cause of infertility and are thought to affect 1 in 10 women. This is when the egg is not released due to hormonal imbalance. Symptoms that show with this condition: excess weight and body hair, acne, mood swings and very few periods or often none at all. A good book that goes into more detail is Dr Adam Laney and Collette Harris' *A Woman's Guide to Dealing with Polycystic Ovary Syndrome*.

- Endometriosis is another condition of hormonal imbalance where there is too much oestrogen. It is a good idea to be screened by an Holistic Practitioner who tests using a Vega machine (or something similar), which screens for genetic inherited toxins, bacteria, viruses, parasites, fungal infections and so forth. Sometimes this form of testing picks up conditions that do not show in conventional blood tests. An example is chlamydia: this bacteria can reside in the fallopian tubes (1 in 10 under the age of 25 are infected). Most people do not even know they have it yet it is one of the known causes of ectopic pregnancy, miscarriage or premature birth. Also gonorrhoea and group B streptococci infections can cause infertility.

- Energy blockages and poor breathing prevent the body functioning properly and is yet another cause of fertility challenges.

- Our own births and how our mothers and fathers nurtured us, have a profound effect on our emotional and psychological make-up. Somewhere buried in the deep recesses of the mind can cause a problem with conception.

Natural therapies can help boost fertility. It is well worth seeing a practitioner.

# Does it make a difference if I have a gap between babies?

Yes, it does. So, if possible, give your body time to recharge and rebuild before conceiving again, ideally a minimum of 18 months to two years.

According to the World Health Organisation, having babies too close to each other slows down the development of the unborn baby as well as growth and mental performance in childhood. The second baby may have a tendency towards a weaker constitution due to less nutrients being available from the mother.

## Case History

Molly came with her two young children, Pippa, aged 4 and Polly, aged 3. Molly had breastfed her oldest daughter and didn't think she could become pregnant while she was doing this. So she was very surprised to find she was pregnant six months after Pippa was born. Now her main concern was how to lose all the weight she had gained. She never had a chance to regain her figure from the first pregnancy, let alone the second. After going through her case history, it was clear that she had many nutritional deficiencies - weak and brittle nails, dry and cracked skin, period pains and PMT, disturbed sleep, sugar cravings and lack of energy. One result of having the children so close together was her flabby, stomach muscles; they never had time to knit back together. However, by addressing her deficiencies and taking Pilates exercise classes, she could certainly improve. This again shows how easy it is to be wise after the event.

# How can the future father of the baby help?

Follow the Wellness Action Plan. Make sure the father is in optimum health, eating a good diet, drinking at least two litres/three and a half pints of water daily and exercising. Taking supplementations as specified in the previous chapter reduces stress and removes harmful substances from his body.

| What to do? | Why? |
|---|---|
| Remove toxic ingredients from the home and work environment | Exposure to oestrogen mimics (female hormone) upsets the male hormonal balance and reduces sperm production. Oestrogen mimics are in some paints, plastics, food packaging, pesticides and cosmetics. |
| Avoid pharmaceutical medication when possible | There are links to infertility and congenital malformations. |
| Stop smoking | Compounds of tobacco damage chromosomes. These are the cells that unite at conception and are the blueprint of a baby. |
| Stop drinking | Alcohol also causes chromosomal defects in sperm, increased risk of birth defects, miscarriage, infertility (80% of male alcoholics are sterile) and impotency. This is because alcohol exposes sperm to acetaldehyde, a by-product of alcohol metabolism which affects the sperm concentration, formation, output, motility and tail formation. Alcohol also lowers testosterone levels, the male hormone. Sperm take three months to form, so it is a good idea to stop drinking four months before you are planning to conceive with your partner. |
| Recreational drugs have to be stopped | Cannabis is linked to reduced sperm count, motility and abnormality, impotence as well as stillbirths and impaired mental functioning. It contains tetrahydrocannabinol, which is similar in chemical structure to testosterone and one spliff lowers testosterone levels and libido for up to 36 hours! |

It takes 90 days to make sperm and the current sperm count levels are declining due to a number of reasons including vitamin and mineral deficiencies, pollution and even mobile telephones carried in pockets. Research by the US Government shows that proportionately a man now produces only one third as much sperm as a hamster!

To end this step, I would like to quote Leonardo da Vinci who discovered that a developing baby "does not breathe because it lies continually in water. If it were to breathe it would be drowned; breathing is not necessary to it because it receives life and is nourished from the life and food of the mother." This is what we are highlighting in a very poignant story about one of my older patients, Mrs Dorothy Brown, as the purpose of this book is to give information and practical advice on how to give a baby the best start. This story leads us from pre-pregnancy to pregnancy.

Dorothy, a small, compact, round faced woman in her early seventies, was a grandmother to eleven grandchildren. Widowed at the age of fifty, her four children, three girls and a boy, were her life and had helped her through the early loss of her husband. After this loss, she went on to lose all three daughters to breast cancer and now her son had prostate cancer. She was at her wit's end wondering why she had passed on such bad genes.

The reason for coming to the practice was because she wanted help with the arthritis in her hands and knees as well as her fluctuating energy levels. She had become the central part of her grandchildren's lives and needed to be healthy and to remain active. She had taken care of herself over the years, eating healthily and never to excess. Counselling had helped her with her grief and she knew that she had done everything possible to help her daughters through their ordeals and had been by their bedside as each one had died.

When I told her about this book, she said she had never considered that anything other than bad genes were to blame. She was unaware that the effects of chemicals, toxins and pollutants in her body or in her husband's sperm could affect the baby. The whole concept of pollution in the womb or of the sperm was new to her. She had always put down the untimely death of her daughters to their genes. We talked more about the possibilities of toxic pollutants, harmful ingredients and overall nutritional health affecting the health of the next generation, as well as the birth process itself.

She said she wished she had known more and with great sadness she said, "please include my story in your book to encourage others to consider these possibilities and to take action early enough to clear themselves of anything harmful that could cause or contribute to the premature death of their offspring."

*"The most threatening aspect of pollution*

*today is intra-uterine pollution".*

**Michel Odent,**
*Primal Health Research*

# Self Assessment Questionnaire
## Are you ready to have a baby?

|  | Yes | No |
|---|---|---|
| **Are you eating, on a daily basis?** | | |
| • unrefined carbohydrates, eg wholemeal flour, wholemeal bread, brown rice? | | |
| • organically grown foods? | | |
| • freshly prepared and home cooked foods? | | |
| • complete proteins, such as pulses and grains especially if you're vegetarian? | | |
| • nuts, seeds and cold pressed oils such as olive oil? | | |
| • food without sugar, salt, preservatives and additives? | | |
| **Are you eating, twice weekly?** | | |
| • fresh meat and chicken organically reared and free of growth hormones and antibiotics? | | |
| • organically produced dairy products made with whole un-homogenised milk? | | |
| **Are you drinking?** | | |
| • 2 litres/3½ pints of filtered water daily? | | |
| • no alcohol and carbonated drinks? | | |
| • no tea, coffee and all other forms of caffeine? | | |
| **Are you?** | | |
| • exercising 2 or 3 times a week? | | |
| • having 10 minutes of fresh air and daylight daily? | | |
| • attending any pilates or yoga classes? | | |

|  | Yes | No |
|---|---|---|
| **Are you taking?** | | |
| • vitamins, minerals, probiotics and essential fatty acids? | | |
| • time-out in the day to relax? | | |
| • sufficient rest time and having enough sleep? | | |
| **Have you eliminated?** | | |
| • smoking and any form of recreational drugs? | | |
| • the contraceptive pill? | | |
| • electro-magnetic pollution, where possible? | | |
| • toxic chemicals from your home, your body and medicine chest? | | |
| **Have you visited?** | | |
| • a dentist for a dental check-up? | | |
| • an osteopath/a chiropractor to assess your spine? | | |
| • an holistic practitioner for a general check-up, including checking if you are free of parasites, genito-urinary infections and allergies? | | |
| • a family planning clinic or switched to natural family planning? | | |

Your aim is to answer every question as *"Yes"!*

Where you have answered *"No"* to any question, refer back to the Step 1 in the Wellness Action Plan for review. For further help visit www.viviencleregreen.com/questionnaire2.

# *Step 3 – Pregnancy*

Going through pregnancy can be wonderful, but all too often it is not. In this third step, my aim is to inform and guide you on this journey, to increase your chances of making it wonderful. Ensure you are in sound physical and emotional shape, have a healthy life-style with the best possible diet, together with the right balance of nutrients and reduce your exposure to harmful chemicals. It is vitally important for both you and your baby's future health. After all you don't want your unborn baby swimming around in polluted waters and dumping a load into a tiny body with all the unpleasant effects this entails. The key, however, is to have belief and confidence in yourself as a woman to be able to give birth naturally according to your primal genetic blueprint. This requires understanding of how the body and mind works - a clear vision, careful planning, as well as reassurance and inspiration from those who have experienced it themselves or helped others to do so. Another consideration at this stage is how to feed your new born baby. As the advantages of breastfeeding by far outweigh all the alternatives, this too needs planning and preparation now to pave the way for a smooth transition for the baby after birth. All this and more is what I have collated in Step 3 - Pregnancy.

Now we come to something that may be more challenging to accept. How our babies are born affects not only their physical health, but emotional health too. If we give birth naturally through the vaginal canal, without medication in labour, our babies receive more natural oxytocin, the behavioural hormone now often called the "love" hormone. Then, if undisturbed bonding occurs between mother and baby in the first "Critical Hour" immediately following the birth, that baby will have an even greater exposure to this hormone. This is nature's way of flooding this newly formed being with a huge capacity to love not only itself, but others too. By interfering with this process, we potentially rob the next generation of their ultimate birthright: Wellness.

Through the use of advanced technology and brain scans, science shows that when a baby is born it is still effectively a foetus, only an external foetus. It is not yet a fully formed human being. If humans were like kangaroos, babies would be carried around in a pouch! The baby's brain and its immune, cardiovascular, digestive and hormonal systems are not yet defined. The mass of neural pathways and connections are waiting to be established. We have a vast amount of science and understanding in this field thanks to the work of a leading childbirth specialist, Michel Odent, who has established the Primal Health Research Data Bank. Our babies' health, even their adult health, is shaped between conception and the first birthday and, if a baby's needs are not met then, a lack of growth literally occurs, especially in the brain.

This "human" part (the orbitofrontal cortex) develops almost entirely after the baby is born. What is more, this does not just happen automatically, it only develops out of the baby's experiences with people, primarily with the mother or main carer. An extraordinary example of this can be seen in recent studies of severely deprived Romanian orphans who had been left alone in their cots all day and cut off from any close bonds with an adult. When examined, their brains literally had a black hole where this part of the brain should have been.

This knowledge helps us understand the importance of the baby's relationship with its mother, known in the psychotherapy world as "attachment." This relationship becomes a reference point for all future relationships – it is the foundation of "emotional" stability. Without such stability illness can occur, for example, studies show that 72% of cancer patients had a difficult relationship in their formative years with at least one of their parents.

Another consideration at this stage is how to feed the newborn baby. As the advantages of breastfeeding far outweigh all the alternatives, this must be planned in advance in order to pave the way for a smooth, bonding transition for the baby after birth. All this and more is what I have covered in this next step.

# I have done a pregnancy test from the chemists and it is positive. What do I do now?

From now on everything you do to your body will affect your baby. There is no need for tests at this stage. In fact you can wait 3 months before going to your GP and you have time to get used to being pregnant. Hopefully, you are putting into practice everything suggested in the Wellness Plan and you will be feeling confident in your body's ability to work effectively.

In summary, you need excellent nutrition. This means eating organically grown and unprocessed fresh food, salads and raw foods at every meal for their enzyme content. Eat garlic, onions, eggs, seeds, nuts, green leafy vegetables, bananas and carrots. Wash all fruit and vegetables with water containing a tablespoon of cider vinegar, as this helps to remove some of the toxins on the outside. Eat oily fish at least twice weekly (especially organic salmon, sardines, mackerel and herrings). To season, use fresh herbs and garlic (strengthens the immune system). Drink at least 2 litres/3 and half pints of filtered or glass bottled water daily and avoid all refined carbohydrates such as white flour, white bread, white pasta and white rice (empty foods devoid of nutrition and act like glue in the intestines). Stay away from any hydrogenated fats often found in processed foods as these block the metabolic pathways of the vital essential fatty acids such as those found in oily fish, nuts and seeds. Supplementing the diet with vitamins, minerals, essential fatty acids and probiotics is a must.

Avoid all the toxins from both the external and internal environments e.g. beauty products, sunscreens, bathroom and household cleaning products.

Avoid breathing in traffic fumes and, when at the petrol station, don't breathe in the smells. Animal studies show that sperm of male rats exposed to toxic substances can affect their offspring, so even a father's exposure of toxic substances can affect your unborn baby.

Be aware of heavy metal contamination which can cause problems.

• Mercury - the UK Food Standards Agency advises women to limit their consumption of tuna to no more than two medium size cans or one fresh tuna steak per week and to avoid shark and sword fish. Avoid any exposure to mercury from dental work.

• Lead - causes poor sperm quality and traces have been found in the placentas of some mothers who have given birth to still born babies or where there has been spina bifida or brain damage. Lead can be found and avoided as follows: If working with or sanding old paint, wear a mask, drink purified or glass bottled water, use organic food to avoid lead carrying pesticides, similarly, switch to safer brands of cosmetics.

• Aluminium – is often found in antiperspirants, antacids, aluminium cookware and foil.

• Cadmium - found in cigarette smoke either directly or passively and increases the rate of miscarriage and embryo defects.

Recent scientific research shows that pregnant women using regular shampoo brands could be harming their unborn babies. This is due to the chemical MIT (methylisothiazolinone) found in many popular shampoos, which can affect the development of nerve cells, preventing one cell communicating to another (Pittsburgh University). Unfortunately, safety groups in the UK say there is no firm evidence that it can cross the placenta and go into the circulation of an unborn baby. Let's not wait for that view to change we can take precautions and use products that comply with the Cancer Prevention Coalition.

Allergies are on the increase. According to Dr Michael Radcliffe, one of our leading allergists, 35% of the population are now affected. What is interesting for the purposes of this book is that an infant whose parents both have allergies has a 1 in 2 risk; an infant with 1 parent who has allergies has a 1 in 4 risk; an infant whose parents have no family history has a 1 in 10 risk. By following the Action Plan in Step 1 and by taking the additional nutritional supplements in this Step, parents reduce these risks.

## What happens physically to my body during pregnancy?

Once the sperm has fertilised the ovum and conception has occurred, the egg divides into two. One half becomes the embryo and the other the placenta, the organ that feeds and nourishes the baby. These two are connected by the umbilical cord. All this occurs in a woman's womb (uterus), which is quite an amazing membranous, muscular and nearly transparent bag. At the bottom of this bag is a tight band of muscles known as the cervix which remains tightly closed until labour begins, then the cervix thins and is pulled back out of the way to allow the baby into the birth canal. The cervix is sealed during pregnancy with a plug of thick mucus. When this is expelled around the time of the birth (a show), it is tinged with blood giving it a reddish or brownish colour. The uterus is a small organ roughly shaped like a pear and it grows and expands to the size of a large watermelon to accommodate the ever-increasing size of the baby, the placenta and the fluid. The top of the uterus rises above the lower rib cage pushing the stomach higher than its usual position. What is so amazing is that this increase in size happens gradually so that the rest of the body is able to adjust to this extra load. This explains why we sometimes feel twinges, aches and pains in our muscles and ligaments.

# What vitamins and minerals are advisable to take in pregnancy?

The only routine medical advice given is to tell pregnant women to take 400 mcg of folic acid, which helps prevent neural tube defects such as spina bifida. It is only necessary a month before and for the first 5 weeks after conception.

As already discussed in the Wellness Action Plan, the necessity for supplementation is very important but, to be frank, if after reading this book you go off with shopping list in hand to your local High Street, then you are most likely wasting your time. High Street chemists, supermarkets and so-called health food chains usually sell cheap proprietary/own label brands, the content of which is totally ineffective. It is best to seek professional advice or visit my website for updated information. This is what I generally recommend in the practice:

- Ante natal formula – a general formulation for pregnancy;

- Liquid vitamin and mineral formulation – in an easily assimilated form;

- Vitamin C, 500 mg twice daily;

- Echinacea formula – for immunity;

- Hawaiian Noni Juice – a super fuel for the immune system;

- Essential Fatty Acid, providing 400 mg EPA 200 mg DHA and 200 mg GLA – essential in pregnancy;

- Probiotic - replenishes stores of good bacteria in the gut;

- Rutin - strengthens the walls of the blood vessels, to help avoid spider veins;

- Rubus (last trimester) - raspberry leaf, nourishes the uterine muscle.

# Why are essential fats so important in pregnancy?

What is vital to understand as a pregnant woman is not how many calories or how much protein you eat (although this is important), but what makes the difference to your baby is the quantity and types of fat molecules consumed. These fat molecules, the essential fatty acids (EFAs), are so vital that books are written on this subject alone! But, for our purposes, we know they are needed for prostaglandins - a system of cell regulation. Prostaglandins regulate blood flow to the placenta. They are the control mechanisms for your baby's nutrition. Enough EFAs will reduce the risk of premature and low weight babies and prostaglandin science suggests that it will also reduce the risk of pre-eclampsia. This is because the human brain is made up of 60% fat and, at birth, the baby's head is already 25% of its adult size whereas its body is only 1/20th. So, the priority amongst humans is to feed the developing brain. This natural phenomenon is what separates us from the animal kingdom.

# So how do we know that we have enough of the right fats to meet the needs of a developing new baby?

The best way is to eat oily fish such as organic salmon, sardines, mackerel and herring. These are rich in EFAs especially DHA (dicosapentanoic acid) and, for those who like biochemistry, DHA is a very long chain 22 carbon 6 double bond polyunsaturated fat belonging to the omega 3 family! This means that the fish oils provide the fat molecules that are essential for brain development, they are pre-formed ready for absorption.

If you are vegetarian (not ideal for pregnant women), then you rely on the parent molecule of the omega 3 family (alpha linoleic acid) from which the body, providing it is healthy, will make the required fat molecule. A chemical process called desalinisation occurs and, for this to happen, the body needs minerals such as magnesium and zinc. Dark green vegetables, nuts and seeds (especially flax seeds) are sources of these oils.

## What interferes or blocks my body's ability to use the EFAs from my food?

Pure sugar blocks the absorption of fatty acids, as does alcohol. It is also very important to avoid foods containing hydrogenated fats. These are processed heat treated oils that contain trans-fatty acids which are blocking agents and cross the placenta and prevent your body and your baby obtaining the good and essential fats.

So avoid all vegetable oils (highly processed, cheap oils) unless they are labelled 'cold pressed' and avoid fish and chips, margarines, all cakes, pastries, biscuits and fast foods that use these oils. Be aware that they can be used in anything from mayonnaise to bread and chocolate. In fact, only buy chocolate made with cocoa butter, which usually means continental chocolate. Most chocolate made in England contains hydrogenated fat.

## I have read about "problems" with vitamin A, can you clarify this?

Vitamin A is vital for healthy cells, too much or too little, is to be avoided. Fat soluble sources that come from fish oils are stored in the body whereas water soluble sources from vegetables are not. Vitamin A that comes from fat soluble sources can cause problems as if, too much is taken, the liver becomes congested and being unable to break it all down, causes toxicity. So it is known in the scientific world as a teratogenic, a substance that can create foetal abnormalities such as cleft lip and cleft palate formation. Equally, too little Vitamin A causes serious malformation such as eye defects. The safety range is a minimum of 2,500 IU (750 mcgs) with the ideal being around 5,000 IU (1500 mcgs). Vitamin A is also found in animal liver so it would be unwise for a pregnant mother to eat liver or liver products. Never eat liver from an animial that is not organically reared.

# What are the most common food cravings in pregnancy?

Chocolate seems to be one of the most common, perhaps due to its magnesium content. Stay away, however, from chocolate containing hydrogenated fat as it blocks the absorption of essential fatty acids, vital nutrients for the baby's development.

Pickled cucumbers are often craved too and, if so, pickle them yourself using cider vinegar, the only one beneficial for the body.

# Are there any tips for morning sickness?

Morning sickness is a bit misleading as it can occur at any time of the day, usually in the first 3 months. Personally, I hardly had any. I had absolutely none in the first 3 pregnancies and just a handful of times in my last, multiple pregnancy. It usually only occurs in women whose nutritional status is below par and it is thought that this may be due to an increase in the hormone HCG (human chorionic gonadotrophin) but is also a "thirst signal" of both the unborn baby and the mother. The hormone is produced by the placenta from the moment of conception and reaches its peak around 9 –10 weeks, declining by 14 –16 weeks. By following the Wellness Action Plan, most women will have very little trouble. If, however, nausea and sickness is a problem, try the following suggestions:

- Increase your water intake throughout the day;

- Always have a glass of water with a slice of lemon on rising;

- Be sure you are taking your liquid vitamin and mineral drink, including aloe vera, noni juices and essential fatty acids;

- Breakfast should include some protein foods such as yoghurt or egg;

- Eat small meals;

- Snack on fruit, nuts and seeds;

- Chew well and avoid drinking water at meals;

- Avoid junk foods, hydrogenated fats, artificial additives and preservatives;

- Stop all tea and coffee - try drinking ginger or peppermint tea.

## *What suggestions do you have for constipation?*

Keeping the bowels moving to eliminate poisons and wastes at least once daily is a MUST. You don't want these poisons to re-circulate back into the blood stream and into your developing baby's. It is, however, quite common in pregnancy for the bowel movements to change as the body adapts and makes room for the womb and baby to grow. Keep up your water intake and do not take laxatives from the chemists because of the risk to the baby. Make sure you are following the nutritional supplementation advice given earlier in this step. There are a number of naturopathic suggestions, some may seem rather strange, but keep an open mind, they work! Here are some suggestions:

- Soak 1 – 2 teaspoons of linseeds in a bowl, cover with water and leave overnight, it will go slightly jelly-like. Eat the whole amount with your breakfast.

- Soak prunes and unsulphured dried apricots overnight and eat these for breakfast.

- Dissolve 1 teaspoon of blackstrap molasses in a cup of warm water and drink first thing.

- Grate one small cooked beetroot into a bowl, add some soaked prunes, sunflower seeds and olive oil and eat for breakfast. Beetroot has laxative properties and is excellent for regulating the bowels. It can also be used raw, grated into salads.

For at least one month, completely eliminate dairy which can cause constipation. Do not be concerned about a lack of calcium as this mineral is better absorbed from other sources, such as green vegetables. Dietary fibre is also increased by eating vegetables, both cooked and raw and from whole grains, especially brown rice.

## *I have heard alcohol is bad for pregnant women. Why is this?*

Alcohol crosses the placenta and enters the baby's blood stream causing an increased risk in miscarriage and birth defects. Studies on foetal alcohol syndrome (F.A.S.) show that too much alcohol consumption by pregnant mothers leads to many birth defects. These include heart murmurs, mild facial deformities, low birth weights, congenital hip dislocations and ear infections leading to deafness, short, fused or angled fingers or toes, as well as mental retardation.

Dr Woollam, a Consultant for the World Health Organisation and also a researcher for environmental toxins, states "No alcohol during pregnancy is the only safe limit." If your doctor or midwife advises you that 7 units are safe, they are ill informed.

Studies at Queen's University in Belfast show that even tiny amounts of alcohol, like 4 glasses a week, affect the baby's brain, attention spans and academic performance in school. Even the Bible, written long ago, warns Samson's mother in Judges 13: "You are going to conceive and have a son. Now see to it that you drink no wine or other fermented drink."

Luckily most women do not enjoy alcohol during pregnancy. Just make sure you do not drink as a matter of habit or force yourself for social reasons.

# What homeopathic remedies are advised?

Homeopathy is a very effective way of desensitising hereditary factors that come from previous generations. They are known as "miasms" of which there are five. The pregnant woman carries not only her family's 'miasms' but also her husband's through his sperm. So it is ideal to desensitise them.

See a Homeopath who understands this need and can work with the following protocol recommended by a leading homeopath and naturopath in this field, Martine Faure Alderson. Your regime should include the antidotes for the 5 inherited miasms and should be treated strictly in the following order: Psorinum, Syphilinum, Tuberculinum, Medorrinum and Carcinocin. Every 6 weeks one miasm can be treated out over 2 to 3 day periods using a potency ranging from c30 to c200.

# What do I do if I have a problem with my teeth while I am pregnant?

Ideally, do not interfere with your teeth during pregnancy. If you need a filling, don't have a silver (amalgam) one – opt for a white one instead. Amalgam contains different metals including mercury, a toxic metal, which can seep into both you and your baby's blood stream and can cause mental and physical problems. If you find that jewellery gives you a rash, especially cheap earrings, then you may well have an allergy to nickel, perhaps due to metal filings. Ask your dentist to use a temporary measure that can be dealt with after you have finished breastfeeding. Sometimes a pregnant woman's gums bleed and this is a sign of inflammation often due to vitamin and mineral deficiency. Double check that you are not using toothpaste with sodium lauryl sulphate which aggravates this condition. Look on the box for the list of ingredients. And on no account should you use a mouthwash that contains alcohol.

# What exercise should I do in pregnancy?

It is good to exercise in pregnancy but not excessively. Too much creates free radical activity that causes cellular damage. Pilates, Yoga, swimming and walking are recommended. Finding a suitable teacher is a must. If you haven't started Pilates before coming pregnant then you have to wait till after the first three months. With yoga, especially a Birthlight yoga teacher, you can start any time. When swimming, make sure you are in a good position. Swim with your face in the water (use goggles) so that you do not crush your neck by arching it backwards. Swimming on your front makes lots of space for the unborn baby. I loved an unusual stroke, back crawl arms with breaststroke legs – a suggestion from my Alexander technique teacher, Glynn MacDonald. A bit strange maybe but this combination prevents straining the lower back. Do not kick with straight legs towards the end of pregnancy for this reason.

# Good posture makes a huge difference to having a great pregnancy and an easier birth. What do I need to know?

Be aware of your posture. Notice what position you are when you go about your daily activities, e.g., while sitting, standing, reading, watching TV or driving. Avoid at all costs, slouching, especially the couch potato position and crossing your legs! Lengthen your spine and neck, relax your shoulders and gently nod your neck to see if it is free. Do this right now. Once you feel you have straightened up and are relaxed, take your hand and place it on the back of your neck. Notice if it feels straight. Is it bent forwards or backwards? Straighten up if it is not. Now place your hand on your lower back and see if there is hollow or not. Repeat as before. Being aware of your posture does not always mean that you are in the most comfortable position. Bad habits become comfortable!

A baby will find the best position for itself according to the space you give it. By being aware of your posture, you will encourage your baby to be in a better position for birth.

The squat position is extremely helpful for the birth itself, so practise this at home. Stand with the feet hip width apart, feet parallel and squat down so as to stretch. Doing this throughout the pregnancy helps. It is also a lovely feeling doing this naked as you feel the bump of your tummy on your thighs – a very special feeling! Make a habit of squatting morning and evening when you clean your teeth so that this becomes part of your daily routine.

## What do I need to think about when it comes to Planning The Birth?

We may not always have the opportunity or foresight to plan being pregnant but, once so, we know that birth and motherhood follows. The importance of understanding each stage before we arrive there makes a huge difference. For example, knowing how the body and mind works can help us to make decisions about how and where we are to have the baby long before it arrives. In the same way, looking into the pros and cons of natural versus medically assisted childbirth and breast versus bottle feeding can empower us to make informed choices. In my practice, I ask pregnant mothers to consider where they are going to have the baby. Is pregnancy a healthy function of the body? Yes, is the most common response. Are hospitals for sick people? Yes, is again the common response. So does it make sense to go to hospital, with all that this entails, when you are well and going through a normal bodily function? No, not really! So it is well worth looking at the possibilities of home birth or going to a birthing unit or centre. Do not assume that birth is an illness which requires surgery!

I also recommend that pregnant mothers prepare for birth and motherhood, both physically and mentally. Physically by joining for example, a yoga or active birth class and mentally by becoming the watcher of your mind, notice your thoughts and concerns and write them down so that you can let go of the negative ones and replace these with positive ones. What goes on in the subconscious mind has a huge effect on the eventual outcome, even your own birth memories will have a bearing.

When it comes to childbirth and breastfeeding, we do, however, have a helping hand from nature as our body is programmed to adapt for pregnancy and birth; finding out more about how the body and mind work makes each stage easier. With knowledge and understanding, you can make informed choices when it comes to the birth plan. However you give birth will impact your mind, body and spirit and your emotions, for not only the rest of your life but, the rest of your baby's too. Never be afraid to communicate clearly your desire for a natural birth to your midwife/doula/obstetrician/doctor who will be only too willing to support you in every way.

# Twelve Good Reasons to have a Natural Childbirth

## Baby

1. Better for the baby's physical, mental and emotional health;

2. No painkillers and anaesthetics in the mother's bloodstream so baby can latch on and suckle straight away – helps with bonding;

3. The cranial bones are massaged through the birth canal which stimulates the brain and ensures its development;

4. Coated in the mother's vaginal fluids which protects the baby from infection and bacteria as it comes out of its sterile womb environment into the world of microbes;

5. Bathed in love hormones (oxytocin) at birth and in the first hour of afterwards when there is a rush of oxytocin, flooding the baby with love, joy and euphoria;

6. Opportunity for skin contact stimulating the nerve endings.

## *Mother*

1. Gravity can assist the mother in a natural active birth;

2. Avoiding surgery means the mother has a better chance of walking after the birth or within 24 hours so no need to stay in hospital;

3. No need for episiotomy (cutting of the muscle) and less damage to female genital area;

4. Hormones flood the mothers body giving her natural painkillers and feelings of love, joy and euphoria;

5. Emotional bonding between mother and baby that leads to happier motherhood;

6. A mother regains her figure more quickly.

# How can I use my mind to the best advantage for my developing baby and myself?

Western Philosophy preaches that our minds and bodies are separate from each other and it assumes a total separation between mind and body and that thoughts and feelings do not matter when it comes to our health. So when something goes wrong with the body, we are taught to believe that pharmaceutical medicines or surgery will be necessary and that what goes on in our thinking process is ignored. Yet the cause may be a negative emotion. However, we now know that what we think generates molecules of emotion in our blood stream and these tiny molecules go to every cell transporting this emotion through the whole body and even to our babies via the mother's placenta. As a result of this our babies will be experiencing our feelings, too.

Read or revisit the question "How does thinking affect Wellness?" in the first Step, which gives a basic understanding. With awareness, we can choose what we think about. However, to do this we need to focus on goals in our life and to have a favourable outcome we need to take some steps to do this. Picture your baby enjoying life in the lovely, safe, watery cocoon of your womb. As it grows and develops, it enjoys all the different movements that you make as you go about your daily routine. The growing baby loves hearing you talk and sing. Hearing is one of the first senses to develop and your voice is one of the most reassuring noises your baby hears on arrival into this world. Imagine that you are in a wonderful state of being and see yourself happy and calm with a permanent smile on your face enjoying your changing shape. Life can throw up challenges from time to time and the best way to deal with them is to come back to the picture of your mind:

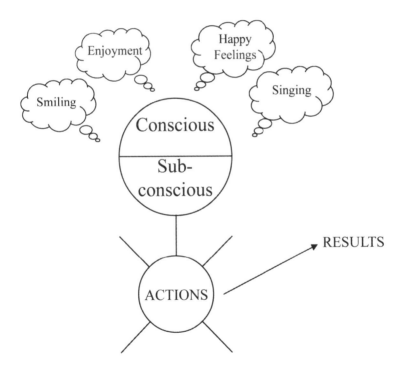

Orderly thinking in your conscious mind leads to order in your body.

Believe in yourself as a mother who is able to give exactly what her developing baby needs. Be very clear in your thinking - orderly thinking in your conscious mind will lead to order in your emotions and order in your body and this applies to the baby too. This gives you sanity, peace and health.

Write out on a piece of paper a positive affirmation in the present tense which feels right to you. Read this twice daily on rising and before retiring. Here are some ideas:

*I trust in the laws of nature and procreation,*
*my baby thrives in every way, I am at peace.*

*I rejoice in being pregnant, I love carrying this*
*growing baby and I love my body and mind.*

*I am a strong, healthy, capable woman who loves*
*and approves of herself in every way.*

*I give thanks to the Creator for my being able*
*to be the home for this developing soul.*

*I love and approve of myself in every way and have complete trust in*
*my body and mind's ability to give the best to this developing embryo.*

These are some ideas. Experiment with different sentences until you gain a feeling, a knowing sensation, that you have hit the right wording for you!

# *If I am very stressed or become emotionally upset, will it affect my baby?*

Studies show that the emotional state of a woman can influence the well being of her child. For example, extreme fear can reduce the blood flow to the womb/uterus and the placenta, which affects the unborn baby's growth. If a lot of adrenaline is made this will increase testosterone levels, (the male hormone) which will adversely affect the baby's hormone levels, its heart rate and blood pressure. So it is important that all those people around a pregnant woman should protect her and surround her with positive emotions. According to Odent, "The primary preoccupation of those who live with or meet a pregnant woman is to protect her emotional state." He has one rule: "Be happy and eat well!"

It is a good idea to have simple ways of calming yourself down. Life often becomes stressful and some days can go out of balance. A useful technique that Louise Hay suggests is to say to oneself a simple sentence repeating it 3 times, like a mantra: "Everything is alright in my world, out of this only good will come." Close your eyes and breathe calmly through your nose visualising the colour blue and then imagine the sea, this will automatically calm you down.

Visualisation is enormously powerful. We think in pictures and have a constant screen running in our minds. Let's try an experiment now: If I say don't think of an elephant, you can't help but do so. Now it is just a question of which way is it facing? The actual written word "elephant" does not flash up in your mind. Then think of your home or your partner or the supermarket and again another picture will flash up. It is as if we have a constant screen in our minds with a permanent show running all the time. The modern way of life has sped up the frames on the film, everything moves more quickly and often we are unprepared, this leads to uncontrolled stress. Meditation is a great way of slowing down the speed of the film and therefore an ideal method of lowering stress levels.

Here is a simple meditation:

Come back to the present moment and concentrate your five senses on your surroundings.

What can you see? What can you hear? What can you smell? What can you taste? What can you feel?

This just brings your mind fully to the present moment. Slowly breathe out, exhaling every bit of breath and then slowly breathe in. Now repeat this but this time as you breathe out, imagine whatever has been bothering you, disappearing and as you breathe in, imagine white light going in through your nostrils and filling your whole body and mind. Instantly you will feel like a completely different person. The stressful moment was just a figment in your mind!

Then imagine yourself floating in a warm sea with blue skies above and not a care in the world, allow yourself to feel the warmth of the sun penetrating your skin removing all muscular tension and wallow blissfully in the moment knowing you have no cares or responsibilities. Then come back to the present moment keeping that sense of positivity inside you to help you through your day. To obtain a relaxation CD go to www.viviancleregreen.com/relaxcd

## *Does the baby's emotional attachment to the mother begin during pregnancy?*

Yes. Attachment, the bond made by a mother with her child, begins the moment a baby is conceived and the unborn baby attaches itself to the wall of the mother's womb. All her thoughts and imaginings about the unborn child are transmitted to the developing embryo. The ideal is to raise a securely attached child which means that the first relationship this baby experiences is with his or her mother and if that bonding (attachment) is secure then this will create a pattern of good relationships with other people for the rest of his or her life. This first relationship is the first entry into the child's database, so to speak and he or she will use it as a base measurement. So the more we can do at this stage, the better. Of course, if there is a problem there are therapies to remove any negative programming, so not all is lost! However, as we are talking in this book about giving our babies the best start in life then we need to consider this important aspect.

How we think generates positive or negative thoughts. A simple exercise to create awareness of this is to keep a diary a few days or even a week recording everything we say to ourselves. This can be a very illuminating exercise and it shows us what is going on in our minds. Then we can start to replace positive thoughts instead of negative ones and reprogram our subconscious mind.

The first six weeks are essential for establishing a good relationship with the new baby. We have to remind ourselves that this first relationship sets a pattern for all future relationships with people for life.

## *What can I expect from my GP?*

GPs (General Practitioners) are used to dealing with disease and ill health and being pregnant is a natural healthy function of the body. So the only thing a GP can do is to detect any big genetic abnormalities. Routine ultra sounds do not serve much purpose. It is far better to have one on demand than just for the sake of it. The best advice a doctor can give is to reassure the expectant mother that she will feel different being pregnant but feeling different is normal. Be happy and eat well! It is not a good idea to fill the expectant mother's mind with negative and worrying information, especially if false readings are given.

A pregnant mother is not obliged to have a routine scan at 12 weeks. Ask your doctor: "What do you expect from this scan?" He may reply, "I want to know exactly when you conceived." To which you can reply: "Is it really necessary?" Or of course he may say that he wants to check that the baby is ok. It is at this stage that you have to ask yourself whether you would take any action if there were to be a problem. If, for example, at 32 weeks you were told that the baby was growing normally but too slowly, what would you be able to do other than leave well alone and follow the maxim "Eat well and be Happy"?

# Are we sure that exposure to ultrasound is perfectly safe?

Various studies have been done, one study concluded that foetal growth was restricted in the early stages. Two other Scandinavian studies showed that ultrasound modified the right and left-brain hemispheres and that use at the beginning of pregnancy was more serious than at the end. Another randomised control study on the use of ultrasound scans, published as long ago as September 16, 1993 in the New England Journal of Medicine, a highly respected and very serious medical journal, concluded that it was better if they were used on demand, as regular screening did not affect the final outcomes.

Looking at it from a different viewpoint one can ask the question as whether it is invasion of the newly forming human being's privacy. Perhaps it was intended that this was a very private time for the mother and baby and that shining bright lights into the womb at this stage might be disturbing.

# What do I need to know about my due date and how accurately can it be predicted?

A developing baby needs 9 months in the womb. In the U.K. the due date is calculated from the last period. This is really a rule of thumb or a rough guide, not a date to etch in stone.

Women's cycles are not always regular 28-day cycles, sometimes they are longer, shorter or even irregular. After coming off the contraceptive pill, it takes a while for the cycles to regulate. So work out, if you can, when you conceived the baby and then compare the date with the one you have been given. If you cannot remember exactly when the baby was conceived, go back to the time when you suddenly couldn't tolerate smoking or being in a hot room or having a craving for something. This is usually 14 days after conception. Odent calculates 41 weeks from the date of the last period. He finds this to be a more accurate time frame.

No one can possibly predict exactly when a baby should be born. In a healthy pregnancy where a mother is aware of what she can do to look after herself and consequently the developing baby, there is no reason why the baby will not be born when it is ready and when you and the baby are ready together. Then allow the birth process to happen the way nature intended. You can always tell your midwife or obstetrician that you want to wait for spontaneous labour to occur.

One very good piece of advice is to tell people an approximate date. It becomes very disconcerting when everyone, from family to friends, starts ringing you up wanting to know when the baby is coming as this stimulates the stress hormones and slows down the start of labour.

## What do I need to know about the routine antenatal tests such as iron levels?

It is very important to remember that the emotional state of a pregnant woman is a priority. Any negative information has not only an adverse effect on the mother but also on the developing baby, as the chemical messengers (hormones) will circulate from the mother's blood stream through the placenta to the baby's.

Routine antenatal tests need to be understood. One of these tests is a blood test to check for haemoglobin/ iron levels (red pigment in the blood). Many people are unaware of some very important published studies on the subject. All we need to know is that when pregnant the mother's blood volume increases by 40–50% so the blood becomes more dilute and iron levels are lower. The up to date thinking on this subject is that the ideal levels in pregnancy are around 9-9.5. This is not a sign of anaemia and if you are advised to take iron supplementation point your doctor or midwife to these studies. If your iron levels do not drop below 10.5 then there is an increased risk of premature birth. If this is the case, increase your water levels (2 –3) litres/31/2-5 pints a day and reduce your consumption of iron rich foods such as liver. If for some reason you need to take extra iron, never take it on its own as it inhibits the absorption of zinc, a very important mineral in growth.

Sometimes women are told they can't have a home birth due to their low iron levels and the risk of excessive bleeding after the birth. This is inaccurate information, there will be more blood lost, however it is more dilute than normal anyway.

Bleeding after labour can seem frightening, especially if you lose a large quantity of blood, but if you know that your blood is 40% more dilute than normal, then it does not seem as frightening. Drink oxygenated water and liquid minerals throughout the pregnancy and your body will restore its levels to normal very quickly.

## Is it likely for my blood pressure to increase during pregnancy?

Yes, it may increase and is to be expected as a healthy symptom. This is very different to blood pressure elevated due to cardiovascular disease. Studies as far back as the 1980s show that women whose blood pressure increased towards the end of pregnancy had very good outcomes (Primal Health Research, volume 10, 2002).

## How can I prevent stretch marks on my boobs and tummy?

Massage daily with almond oil into which has been added essential oil of tangerine. Use the ratio of 20mls of almond to 10 drops of tangerine (20ml: 10 drops). Stretch marks occur due to mineral, vitamin and essential fatty acid deficiency so following the nutritional suggestions will also help to prevent them.

With regard to breasts, make sure you wear a comfortable bra and as they increase in size during the pregnancy, buy a bigger one. There is no reason to end up with stretch marks.

# What essential oils are beneficial in pregnancy?

Essential oils should never be taken internally and should be mixed with a cold pressed vegetable oil such as almond, avocado, or coconut oil. Each oil has specific healing properties:

**Tangerine** - the best oil of all for pregnancy, with a general harmonising effect on the mind and body and good for preventing stretch marks (see previous question),

**Orange** - fortifies and is a tonic for the nervous system,

**Neroli** - calming for the nervous system,

**Lemon** - good for high blood pressure and veins,

**Lavendern** - good for burns, immune boosting, stress, insomnia, tension, aches and pains, fluid retention and skin irritations,

**Chamomile** - alming and soothing for the skin and digestive system,

**Cajuput, eucalyptus, pine** - good for colds, sinusitis and flu.

# What can be done to prevent myself tearing during the birth?

The skin that connects the vaginal opening to the anus is known as the perineum and during pregnancy, this area becomes more elastic in preparation for the birth. To increase the elasticity, this area can be massaged in the last 3 months with almond oil and then very gently stretched with the fingers. The idea is to stretch the entrance to the vagina as wide as possible. This can be done towards the end of pregnancy 2 or 3 times. You can involve the father of the baby with this!

# Is there a good protocol to be taken to help with the delivery?

The homotoxicological (progressive homeopathy) protocol is very effective. These preparations come from Heel in Germany (www.viviencleregreen.com/heel).

- **Traumeel** - 5-6 tablets, for 1-2 weeks before delivery and 2 weeks after delivery.

- **Coenzyme and Ubichinon compositum** - 1 ampoule twice weekly for 1 month prior and after delivery.

- **Cimicifuga-Homaccord** - for nervous and skeletal systems. Also good for postpartum depression - 15 drops two times per day, for 2 weeks before delivery and for 1 month post delivery.

- **Aconitum-injeel S** - 1 ampoule per day 3 days before due date or after water breaks, for fear and pain.

# I have heard of pre-eclampsia. Is it dangerous?

This is a life threatening disease to both the mother and the baby, but it is very rare. Accurately diagnosed eclampsia rates are 2-3 per thousand and this tends to occur only in developing countries. High blood pressure readings are often confused with this disease, in the same way as a headache could be with a brain tumour. Do not assume the worst from common symptoms, it is diagnosed by two specific tests.

1. Increased blood pressure.

2. A urine test measuring protein – this necessitates collecting samples over a 24-hour period (not just a single collection). Once tested in the lab, the presence of more than 300mg of protein over the 24 hour period, assuming there is no urinary tract infection, would indicate eclampsia.

Confusion occurs and some women become frightened unnecessarily when their blood pressure goes up and a single test stick shows there is protein in the urine. Make sure you have a proper test as described above. It is reassuring to know that an increase in blood pressure can be a good sign, as it means that there is an enhanced arterial blood flow to the placenta, i.e. healthy placental activity.

Odent's own interpretation is that this is maternal foetal conflict. The unborn baby is asking more of the mother than she can do. One document shows that the levels of maternal unsaturated fats are very low and Odent suggests that the mother does not have enough essential fatty acids to feed the brain of her developing baby. Good nutrition with adequate intake of oily fish is a good preventative measure. Studies show there is no pre-eclampsia in the Seychelles where, on average, a pregnant woman eats 22 meals a week of sea fish. We must never forget that large brains in humans need Omega 3 essential fatty acids.

## Another symptom of which to be aware – HELPP Syndrome

It is a disease that tends to occur at the end of a first pregnancy. Suddenly out of nowhere, stomach pains occur that are not the usual digestive ones. This is a sign to immediately contact your doctor or midwife as this can be a sign of HELPP syndrome (Haemolysis elevated liver enzymes low platelet counts.), a condition related to pre-eclampsia.

## A friend was told she had gestational diabetes. What is it; can I prevent it; what do I do if I have it?

A glucose tolerance test is given to see if the mother has elevated glucose in her blood after consuming certain sugars. However, this can be a transitory physiological response (i.e. it occurs in a healthy pregnancy) and should not be confused with diabetes, which can be a serious condition.

According to Odent and recent research, there are no evidence based medical studies to support this so-called "gestational diabetes". And, if medication such as insulin is prescribed, ostensibly to lower the blood sugar levels, it will actually restrict foetal growth with potentially fatal consequences. Unless the mother is truly diabetic, a glucose tolerance test showing higher levels of sugar in the blood simply means that the woman has an unbalanced diet with excess sugar! (Primal Health, volume 12, no 1).

All pregnant women should avoid pure sugar, soft drinks and sodas and eat complex carbohydrates, such as whole-wheat pasta, whole-wheat bread and brown rice. This avoids the ups and downs in the blood sugar level which places such a strain on the digestive system and gives such erratic energy. A useful way of assessing the absorption rate of foods is to use the glycaemic index (GI), or better still, the glycaemic load (GL). These indices show how fast blood sugar is raised by different foods.

It really does not matter which system is used as it all comes back to eating a healthy un-refined diet as laid out in the Wellness Action Plan.

Exercise is also important to blood sugar levels balance. You should do a certain amount of physical activity every day, even if it's only half an hour's walk.

## *My tummy goes really hard sometimes but it is not painful. Why is this?*

This is quite normal and is due to the tummy (uterine) muscles contracting, they are known as Braxton-Hicks contractions. The body is very cleverly designed! It knows to train for a marathon and that the uterine muscles need a regular workout and it does all this quietly, without the mother realising. From time to time, when placing your hand on your abdomen, you will feel hard and rigid, but it is not painful in any way. Each contraction lasts from 30 – 60 seconds in a series that lasts for as little as 10 minutes and as long as 60 minutes. It is a very good sign.

# Is there anything I can do to prevent having an underweight or premature baby?

Yes! It comes back to understanding the basic needs of a pregnant woman from an emotional as well as a nutritional point of view. From the emotional point of view, do not allow situations to upset you, don't look at books, magazines, videos or TV that create fearful pictures in your mind. This will have a biochemical reaction in your body and can be passed through your blood to your developing baby. Studies show that extreme stress in a pregnant woman shuts down the blood flow from the mother to her baby, which can cause all sorts of problems.

From a nutritional point of view, have plenty of essential fatty acids especially DHA (dicosopentanoic acid) from oily fish. Studies show that premature births were as low as 1.9% in one group of mothers who regularly eat fish and as high as 7.1% in another who do not. The same applied to low weights at birth.

Recent understanding shows the importance of feeding the brain. Imagine a starving human being in times of famine with a big head and a thin body. This demonstrates the priority in man is to protect the brain.

# Is breastfeeding best for my baby?

Absolutely. Two of the principle long-term effects of breastfeeding are disease prevention and higher immunity. A baby in the womb is completely sterile, but at the moment of birth it enters the world of microbes/bacteria. Did you know that there are no microbes in the intestine of the unborn baby, but 24 hours later, there are billions and trillions? The intestine is wide open to foreign proteins viruses, toxins and germs, but the act of vaginal birth and the baby's first liquid secretion (colostrum) from its mother's breast each, in turn, protect the baby from the outside and the inside. Colostrum contains antibodies, protein, nutrients and growth factors, so it suppresses any infection. It is nature's miracle food.

Racehorse breeders know that a foal deprived of colostrum will never be a champion! Even if there are cases of toxins or chemicals in the mother's milk resulting from her own internal pollution, the advantages of breastfeeding far outweigh any disadvantages. Rates of child survival in third world countries show the spectacular positive effects of breastfeeding. Breast is best!

## Benefits to the Baby

- Healthy gut due to beneficial bacteria "bifido",
- Antibodies to help the baby's immunity,
- Hormones and growth factors to help promote growth,
- Brighter and more alert,
- Less likely to be overweight,
- More fat soluble vitamins,
- More alkaline,
- Reduced risks of suffering gastric complaints, ear infections, allergies, diabetes and childhood and adult cancers
- Better eyesight, reduced risks of myopia,
- Protected from hypertension / high blood pressure later in life,
- Stronger jaw muscles and co-ordination in general,
- Healthy bonding/attachment with the mother is vital to all subsequenta relationships in life.

## Benefits to the Mother

- Reduces chances of breast and ovarian cancers,
- Wonderful bonding with the baby,
- Stimulates the uterus to contract to its pre-birth size,
- Excess weight rapidly disappears,
- Very easy to carry around and always at the right temperature!

# Will my opinions about breastfeeding affect my results?

Yes. How we think about breastfeeding will dictate our results. When I first fed my first child, I remember going for my six-week check up to my Naturopath, John Sugarman. He told me that I should feed Sophie for six months. I had no idea that you could feed a baby only breast milk for so long. It came as a real surprise and I went home in the car saying to myself over and over again "six months"! As I had done it for a few weeks I thought to myself, "I suppose I just keep going!" Now at least I knew this when it came to feeding the twin girls and I wanted to be able to give them what I had given to the other three children, the best start, so I set out to feed them exclusively for six months. I never could have done it if I hadn't set the goal and had the desire to do so before they were born and it was worth everything.

Many mothers have preconceived ideas or negative opinions that prevent them breastfeeding. On further examination, usually they don't believe they are capable of doing so or that it will spoil their figure or restrict their movements. These misconceptions are easily overcome when speaking to mothers who have done so, myself included. Every woman is capable, it is nature's blueprint; the breasts change in pregnancy in preparation for feeding and will go back to their shape afterwards. The ageing process is something else! Finally, breastfeeding makes it easy to travel and go about daily life with the baby. These examples show the power of the mind has a huge bearing on the eventual outcome.

# Now that I know the benefits of breastfeeding and have made the decision in my mind to do so, what can I do during my pregnancy to help make this easier?

First time mothers who have never experienced breastfeeding may be slightly surprised by the sensation of a baby feeding. Most women only touch their nipples when washing and any other touch is usually associated in a sexual way. Actually, when a baby latches on it is a very firm feeling and it is a good idea to toughen up the nipple area by squeezing your nipples quite firmly each day throughout the pregnancy. The father of the baby can also be asked to help here! It is also a good idea to massage the breasts daily. To do this, apply a little almond oil into the palm of your hand, start at the top of your breast and in a circular movement, massage first clockwise 3 times and then anti-clockwise, 3 times, round the outside of the breast. This helps to keep the circulation and lymph system moving and to prevent breast tenderness and stretch marks. The use of nutritional supplements ensures that your body produces the best possible milk supply.

## Can painkillers affect my baby?

The baby will absorb the effects of painkillers and most likely be "dopey" at birth, making breastfeeding difficult to establish. As explained earlier, this blocks the mother's production of natural "feel good" hormones in her milk supply and ultimately in her baby. A baby thus deprived is more likely to turn to chemically addictive substances or narcotics as an adult.

## What about sex during pregnancy?

Enjoy it! It is perfectly safe all the way through pregnancy even to the birth itself.

# What clothes and accessories do I need to buy for the baby before it is born?

Initially the baby will need cotton vests, baby grows, nappies/diapers, a couple of cardigans, a hat and a shawl. It is very tempting to buy lots of things, but the best advice is to buy the minimum at this stage. The most important thing to buy is a baby carrier/sling and probably a car seat. It is far better to carry the baby on you than to push it in a pushchair. You may want a Moses basket for the baby to sleep in or you may decide to have the baby in your bed. Don't be tempted to buy lots of equipment, as it is very easy to stock up on items that will never be used. A changing mat/fold up bag is another must, as is a waterproof and easy to wipe surface for changing nappies/diapers. When it comes to washing the baby, use whatever bathroom facilities you have. It is possible to buy shaped sponges that sit in a bath or the shower tray. Washing a baby in the bath with the mother is very pleasurable, made even more enjoyable if there is someone to take the baby out while you stretch out and enjoy a few moments to yourself!

# What bathroom products do I need to buy for the baby before it is born?

Very little. Cotton wool and water is best to wipe a newborn baby's bottom and then use a liquid soap, perhaps with aloe vera. Avoid products with harmful ingredients as discussed in the Wellness step and only use those recommended by the Cancer Prevention Coalition.

Products to avoid in particular include most talcum powders, baby wipes and commercial baby oils. Use oils for massage that are safe to eat such as almond oil.

To stress the importance of harmful ingredients: a recent royal commission investigated 4000 chemicals and found 66% of them to be toxic and 50% carcinogenic. Talcum powder has the same molecular structure as asbestos, a known cancer-causing agent and there are links with talcum powder and ovarian and testicular cancers. Another chemical compound, DEHP, an oestrogen mimic, has been shown to cause genital abnormalities in male babies, even testicular cancer.

## *I have been told that my baby is in a breech position (meaning feet first) and that I should have it turned at 37 weeks. What should I do?*

At 37 weeks it is a fairly standard procedure now for a mother to be given medication to relax the uterus so that the baby can be turned. There are also non-medical ways to turn the baby such as Chinese medicine using acupuncture and moxibustion. An acupuncture needle is placed on the little toe (bladder meridian) and it is heated with moxibustion. Sometimes these methods are successful and sometimes they are not.

Mary, an easygoing woman in her early thirties had a straightforward pregnancy without any complications. She felt apprehensive about her first birth but not frightened. Her mother had told her that she had been born by caesarean as she had been in a breech position. So when Mary went for her check up at 38 weeks and was told her baby had turned into the breech position, she became very anxious. She discussed the various options and decided to have some acupuncture sessions. To her great relief, she went into spontaneous labour and her baby was facing head down. She had a natural birth which lasted 12 hours, from start to finish. Would the baby have turned without the acupuncture session? Who knows! However, by taking some positive action, it helped Mary to feel positive and prevented her from worrying unnecessarily.

# Conclusion

Planning, preparation, positive thinking and practical tips pave the way for not only a healthy and happy pregnancy but also for the best birth possible and the best start for a new baby.

Now I would like to share another story with you about two mothers with their two-week old babies. One had planned the next stage and the other just lurched along.

Just imagine a new thirty-year-old mother, Stephanie, nursing her baby girl, now two weeks old. This mother is tired but calm and content. She gave birth naturally without any painkillers whatsoever in the birthing unit of her local hospital. "A number of people suggested that I opt for an epidural to avoid any pain from childbirth but I felt that would have been weak on my part and that I needed to do justice to myself as a woman," she said. "Call it pride if you like. But for me it was the driving force to be able to have a natural birth without the use of painkillers." Stephanie followed the Wellness Programme and by maintaining a healthy, wholesome diet of organic foods, she did not put on any excess weight. Now two weeks after the birth, her figure is slim and svelte almost without any signs of pregnancy at all. Her womb is returning back to its normal size AND she does not have any stretch marks on either her tummy or her breasts. Breastfeeding has been very easy for her and she feels that this is largely due to the wonderful bonding she and her baby had after the birth, the "Critical Hour" period.

Now imagine another new mother, Dawn, of a similar age. She is trying to breastfeed her 10-day-old baby, but after the initial suckling, he turned away, miserable and dissatisfied. No milk flow seemed to be coming so Dawn offers him a bottle of formula milk, which he gobbles up. She gave birth with painkillers administered through a fine tube in her spine (epidural). "I had chosen this because everyone I spoke to told me the pain was awful and I don't like pain." What she had not anticipated was that the epidural itself was very painful when it was inserted and that she had a huge amount of pain and discomfort afterwards. Her back was so sore she could hardly walk. "It is not like this for everyone apparently, but I have been unlucky. She also felt cheated because she was in a hazy trance, almost a stupour, during the labour and when the baby arrived she was out of it and did not focus on the "Critical Hour" for bonding. Her baby, a beautiful boy, was so dopey that it had been difficult to breastfeed straight away and already he was receiving formula milk and she hadn't established her own supplies properly. In all probability, breastfeeding was not looking very promising.

These two different scenarios are ones that have been presented to me many times in my clinical experience and it is better to be informed and aware of the long term consequences in advance. Prevention is always better and easier than the cure.

# Step 4 - Birth

So many horror stories and prejudices circulate in our society about labour and birth that it is difficult to believe this is beneficial for both the mother and the baby. TV portrays women in dramas or sitcoms, even adverts, as suddenly experiencing a sharp, excruciating pain and everyone starts rushing around in a panic, with ambulances being summoned. Then, in hospital, labour is treated as an acute illness or injury, is over dramatised and appears to be terribly painful and life threatening. Painkilling anaesthetic is made out to be the magic bullet that takes away all evil. This is so far from the truth, yet the portrayal creeps into our belief systems alongside those of our own mothers or friends and this becomes generally accepted. We must dispel this myth and negative programming and one way to do this is to make sure women who intend to be or who are already pregnant fill their minds with positive stories, accurate information and the belief that babies are meant to be welcomed gently into the world with joy and love.

For this reason I have included some birth stories with key ones from my independent research, carried out for the purposes of this book. I would also recommend the stories by Ina May Gaskin, one of the greatest midwives of our time, in her wonderful book Guide to Childbirth.

In my research, I asked 500 women about their labour and birth experiences, grouping the respondents into 3 categories:

1. Those who had natural vaginal births with no medical assistance,

2. Those who chose to have medical assistance, either before they started or during the birth,

3. Those who had had experiences of both.

The objective of this research was to find out how their births had been, what they wished they had known before and had they had known this, would it have altered their experiences. The results made me even more passionate about writing this book and I have addressed these concerns as well as recounting what some of them said in this next Step 4.

First I would like to tell you Mary's story:

Mary was expecting her first baby. In the early hours, she started to feel mild contractions. She rested in bed and, as daylight dawned, went calmly about her morning routine at home now that she had given up work. She paused from time to time to let a small twinge pass. Eventually, the contractions came more frequently and intensely.

She had decided to have her baby in hospital where there was a birthing unit and had visited it a few times so that she felt familiar with the surroundings. On this particular morning, her husband was able to drive her there and, on arriving, she felt a wonderful air of calmness and quiet efficiency that gave her confidence. She had very little monitoring and was allowed to go into her own space, she used the physio ball to rock through the contractions, which by now were vast surges of energy, clearly her labour was progressing well. There was a birthing pool, but it was in use. However, she didn't feel the need for it anyway.

One of the midwives ran the tap in the sink and she could hear the noise of running water. The lights were dimmed and voices were hushed. In her corner, Mary made a sort of nest with towels and beanbags. At one stage, she pointed to her back so that the midwife could rub it through the contractions, her husband, meanwhile, sat quietly in the corner reading his newspaper. Mary went completely into her own world and only remembers someone saying, "The baby is coming." With three pushes and an incredible feeling of stretching, the baby was born. "It was amazing, euphoric," she said. "I shall never forget this experience!"

The story of her second birth was so completely different. She had contracted genital herpes and was told that she could not have a natural, vaginal birth in case she had an outbreak at the time, risking the baby catching it which might have severe consequences. Mary said that, on reflection, she did not do enough research, she just accepted it. She now knows that it is quite possible to have a natural, vaginal delivery with genital herpes and anyway, a woman's immunity is heightened during pregnancy and outbreaks are very rare. Had there been an outbreak, she would have applied essential tea tree oil that inhibits the infection.

So a day was booked for her to have an elected caesarean. When the day came, she remembers so vividly the drive to the hospital with her husband. They drove in complete silence, there was an air of emptiness, not of expectancy. There was absolutely no thrill of the baby coming, it was all so clinical. "Going in to the coldness of the hospital, putting on a gown, being given the first injection and then being wheeled into theatre was like a nightmare." Everything went well according to the medical team and a beautiful baby boy was delivered. She never even went into labour at all.

Afterwards, when she held her newborn baby she felt few maternal feelings, just a sort of numbness. Only one arm was available to hold the baby but what was so different for her this time was her complete lack of maternal feelings, so the baby was immediately passed to her husband. She was white as a sheet, wiped out by the shock of surgery. Breastfeeding was established, but it did not last for long and very soon her baby was on formula milk.

Her words still ring in my ears: "I felt as if I had been robbed." She had six months of post-natal depression.

Mary said that she could not believe the difference between the two births and she said that if only women knew how wonderful it was to have a natural birth and, in comparison, how cold and joyless it was to have a medicated and surgical birth, they would never choose it. What's more they would fight for their rights. Now that she knows of the long-term consequences to the baby's physical and emotional health, she wished she could turn the clock back.

What others have said taken from my research

This is what a mother, who had had three natural home births using a birthing pool, said "Nothing can prepare you for your first baby – it is an earth shattering experience to let go and allow your body to open. It was a wonderful sensation and incredible to have achieved it. The subsequent births were so much easier; they too gave me tremendous fulfilment."

"I chose natural birth over epidural or elective caesarean as I knew the benefits it would give my child and for reasons of pride. I would have felt weak in character if I hadn't tried and that I hadn't done justice to myself as a woman. The cost also came into it. I didn't want to spend the money that way. I would rather pay for a private room afterwards or for some help when I got home!"

While pregnant with her third child, Jane suffered from one of those awful holiday bugs which not only spoilt her trip but continued when she came home. Naturally she was concerned about the effects on her unborn baby. "I nearly lost him and I have to confess that I did wonder if I would bond with the baby as I had been so ill." The plan was to have an elective caesarean like the previous two but it happened so quickly there wasn't time, her baby was born in the hall before the ambulance even arrived. "It was love at first sight, more than anything else I've ever experienced and it's never waned. Amazing! I never knew I could have that depth of feeling for someone and it's not as though I don't love my husband and other two children, but it is a very deep bond".

Helen had two children. The first one was difficult as she didn't dilate and had to be induced. She felt threatened and pushed into being induced by such comments as her uterus could burst or the baby could be caused distress. She felt her body hadn't performed the way nature had intended it to do it and that she had failed. What's more, she had to stay in hospital for several days because of the pain and now around the incision itself it is still numb and she has no feeling in the area.

Marjorie was told her baby was too big after she had been in labour for only five hours and she was delivered with a caesarean. Had she known how her body was able to adjust to accommodate the size, it would have been different. She subsequently had two more children delivered by caesarean because she was told that as her first baby had been big, the next ones would be too. She says she felt slightly cheated in both cases because although her labour started naturally, she was automatically admitted for surgery even when both babies were a normal size.

Anne was so afraid of the pain that she didn't consider any other options. With the information that the pain of childbirth is altogether different to that of injury and that the body has an ability to manufacture its own pain relieving compounds, she would have had a more open mind.

Rosemary said she used gas and air. She said that it can take over from your own rhythm as you almost lose touch with yourself and it is difficult to gain control again. In her third birth, she lost control so much that she thinks she was close to surgical intervention. But her husband told the birthing team to take it away from her and as a result she had a vaginal delivery.

Other mothers said that they had no idea that their births could either be so quick or so slow. Share your story? www.viviencleregreen.com/ birthstoryclub.

When Gwyneth Paltrow gave birth naturally to her baby, which weighed 9lbs 11ozs, she was quoted as saying that although it was a long labour she focused on her late father, Bruce, and imagined how proud of her he would have been.

In 1950, fewer than 3% of women had Caesarean sections. Nowadays, they make up 25% of the annual 600,000 births in England and Wales. Of this 25%, 7% (about 6,000) of Caesarean sections happen for non-medical reasons and these cost the UK government, the NHS about £25 million more than natural births. Now, in the UK, only 53% of births are natural without any intervention.

Today we have the choice of whether to give birth as nature intended, releasing the many hormones that play a key role in the initiation of birth and even of lactation (breastfeeding), or alternately, to intervene medically with synthetic and chemical hormones, which being unable to cross the blood/brain barrier, do not fulfil the bonding and love hormone role of our own naturally formed hormones. To choose the latter usually relies on substitutes for natural hormones - synthetic oxytocin drip or epidural anaesthesia – or even a surgical birth by caesarean section. Mankind in general does not like pain and many regard childbirth as a pain to be avoided at all costs. But the difference here is that the body is already programmed to make its own painkillers, as well as chemicals that create joy and euphoria and, if allowed to function properly, both the mother and baby come away elated!

Science is unable to replace exactly these natural hormones and synthetic hormones only make the body function at a very basic level, completely bypassing all the feeling-good and euphoric factors.

The rise in caesarean births far outweighs the numbers of emergencies and it has become accepted to choose to have a baby in this way. In the United States, the caesarean section is the most common major surgical procedure. Media and modern day obstetrics brainwash women into believing that this is the better way to deliver a baby, but what is so distressing is how this lowers the opportunity for optimum wellness in both the woman and the baby.

Choosing the way in which to give birth is a major decision in a woman's life. However, so little is understood about how this choice ultimately affects not only herself but her baby too. There are lifelong consequences in the building of foundations and the infrastructure of her baby's mental, emotional and physical performance for its entire life. If the baby receives the abundance of hormones nature intended especially of oxytocin, the behavioural love hormone and bonds with its mother in the first hour of life - the "Critical Hour" - and its emotional as well as its physical needs are met in the first and second years of its life, then this baby will have a greater chance of having a secure, loving attachment to its mother.

This is the baby's first relationship and forms the foundation for all successive relationships. More than that, it will respond emotionally much better to the challenges life inevitably offers up. This is because what we know as the immune, the hormonal and the digestive systems - as well as the brain - are not fully formed until the first year of life.

Key advantages of a natural vaginal delivery without any medication are summarized below:

## For the Mother

- She falls in love with her baby - immediate bonding and easy breastfeeding are established.

- Her figure returns more quickly with no invasive surgery or toxicity from medication. She can even walk out of the delivery room.

- Experience of joy and fulfilment – a truly empowering event.

## For the Baby

- Greater capacity to love, not only itself, but others too, due to the release of hormones from its mother.

- Birth occurs when the baby is ready. When the unborn baby's lungs are fully matured, it releases a hormone (signal) which is picked up by the mother's body.

- Coated and protected by the vaginal fluids as the baby enters the world of germs, bacteria and micro-organisms giving enhanced immunity and better health.

- The baby's head is massaged by the birth canal stimulating its brain and spinal cord.

- A generally more contented baby and easier child to raise.

- Less likely to turn to mood altering and often addictive substances in later life.

For further research please visit the Primal Health Research Centre website and view the studies. An example amassed by Dr Michel Odent, Director of the Primal Health Research Centre, shows that babies exposed to opiates during their mothers' labours are more likely to become chemically dependent adults. In his view, exposure in the womb, however brief, imprints itself on the unborn baby's brain as a situation to which the child and later the adult constantly strives to return. It is a difficult task to erase the dependency that we have imprinted into that child and his descendants for generations to come.

## *I have heard that giving birth is painful.*

This is something that is SO misunderstood. Most people's experience with pain is usually as a result of illness or injury. In this sense, pain is a warning that there is something wrong and that attention must be paid in order to deal with the problem. Since the introduction of painkillers, the Western world is accustomed to taking something that stops the pain. The male world tends to view the pain of childbirth in the same way, as a pain that can and should be avoided.

This is the greatest misconception. Giving birth is a completely different pain to that of injury. It is a pain that you do not want to stop and the more you let go and relax into it, the more you enjoy it. Contractions are no more than surges of energy into the muscle. These muscles are not injured they are just working very intensely. The body makes its own painkilling substances together with feel-good hormones. This gives the most incredible euphoria.

# *Explain the chemical messengers known as hormones that are made during labour and birth.*

Oxytocin, prostaglandins, adrenaline and endorphins are the most important ones. These are chemicals made by the woman to trigger the necessary actions of the body.

- Oxytocin (the love hormone) tells the womb to contract and is the hormone (chemical messenger) that makes the mother and child bond and literally fall in love. Oxytocin is involved in any aspect of love, both men and women release it during orgasm and it is during female orgasm that it stimulates the uterine contractions to help transport the sperm towards the egg. The presence of this love hormone peaks and is the greatest just after natural childbirth that is without administered hormones. The importance of this peak is highlighted when it is linked with the knowledge that oxytocin can induce both the mother's and the baby's behaviour to love each other. When breastfeeding, as soon as the mother picks up the signal that her baby is hungry, more oxytocin is released. Perhaps this is nature's way of making sure that the young survive. A parallel can be made with sexual arousal, which frequently starts before there is any skin stimulation! Then as the baby sucks, the level of oxytocin released by the mother is about the same as during orgasm and goes into the breast milk. So a baby will absorb some of this love hormone via its digestive tract. Studies now show that when we share a meal with companions we increase our level of oxytocin. Surely this pattern designed by nature is critical to our lives throughout.

- Prostaglandins stimulate the opening of the womb (cervix) to soften and thin.

- Adrenaline (the emergency hormone stimulated in fear) can halt labour by suppressing the production of oxytocin. However, a spurt at the very end gives the necessary final burst of energy so that the mother is alert and able to protect her baby as soon as it is born.

- Endorphins are the body's natural painkillers and actually block the sensation of pain. They are also hormones of pleasure. During intercourse both partners release high levels. So the system that protects us against pain is one that also gives us pleasure. During the birth process, the baby itself and the mother release their own endorphins so that in the hour following birth both the mother and the baby are impregnated with opiates. Opiates create a state of dependency so both turn to each other and the beginning of attachment is created. This continues into breastfeeding. When a woman is feeding, her endorphin levels peak every 20 minutes and the endorphins are in her milk too. That is why, after being breast-fed, babies sometimes look as if they are on a high with a glazed look in their eyes!

To be absolutely clear, the pain of childbirth is unlike any other pain we normally experience. It is pleasurable. Rather than wanting it to stop, you want it to keep on happening once you let yourself go and surrender. It gives the most incredible euphoria. Some women have even described it as orgasmic, probably because it is an "out of this world" sensation and experience. I always say to women who are going to have a baby, if it were physically possible I would have it for you, as it is so wonderful!

How we think about birth in the deepest recesses of our minds will affect the outcome. Giving birth is a natural, normal, physiological process. If we understand this process and believe and trust in the hormones to be the key to this process, then birth can be a joyful and enlightening experience. It is very important to examine what is in the deepest recesses. For example, if there is a secret fear of tearing or even dying and it is not voiced, then these emotions may block labour progressing. Sometimes these unwanted fears, which are pushed deeper and deeper in our minds, do not surface until labour itself.

I know from personal experience that if you fight the pain of the contractions/surges of energy during childbirth, it becomes more painful. The moment I started to repeat to myself "let go, let go" and breathe out during the contraction, a wave of release swept over me and the pain seemed to disappear.

Relaxation not only relieves the pain, it allows the body to open up for the baby to glide into this world. Visualising the waves in the sea worked beautifully for me and I just imagined the contraction to be like a wave, a surge of energy and I just went with the flow. We all know how hard it is to fight a wave and how magnificent it is to be carried with it.

## Which part of the body works hardest when a woman is in labour?

Believe it or not, the most active part is the archaic, primitive brain, which releases a complex mixture of hormones. Simply put, whilst in labour, a woman's brain is releasing her own chemicals which take messages to all parts of her body to "open the doors" for the baby to be born. What is often misunderstood is that if the brain's intellectual part (the neo cortex, the one we are using now) is stimulated, it slows the production of these hormones and acts as a brake on the birth process.

So we come to the critical point. A woman in labour must do all she can to switch off her thinking brain to let the process happen as naturally as possible. Just imagine that you are trying unsuccessfully to go to sleep, the last thing you want is the TV playing in the next room, flashing neon lights coming through the curtains, or your partner nudging you with questions every few minutes.

Well, it's just the same when giving birth. There is a need for you to withdraw into your own quiet world where there is silence, low lighting, warmth and privacy. Anybody else nearby must understand the crucial needs for calmness, silence and privacy and emotional security.

We all know that feeling of being watched when we think we are alone and how we become suddenly self-conscious. So, no husband, or partner, or birthing attendant and especially no camera or video should be in sight. Even, electronic foetal monitoring has been found to have the same effect.

It is essential that you are not stressed in any way and that includes being disturbed by those around you, whether it be the husband, midwife, friend or obstetrician (who may be rushing to another birth). If someone's adrenaline levels are high, it is very contagious and you will soon feel it. This all goes back to basic survival when, in an emergency, our bodies react instantly in the "fight and flight" pattern; our hearts race, blood rushes to our limbs and energy is released as the body receives the message that it is not safe to deliver the baby and puts the process on hold until the coast is clear.

## How does my body work in labour?

Enormous amounts of physical changes and months of preparation have occurred by the body in preparation for this great event. During the last few days of pregnancy, the cervix (the tight band of muscles that closes the uterus) softens and thins to allow the baby to pass through the birth canal. This is known as "ripening" and is due to hormones called prostaglandins.

Gradually the first stage of the birth process begins. Intensified signals pass between the mother and baby so that their bodies work together and, when both are ready, the dance of the birth movements begins. It starts with the baby tapping on the cervix with its head or sometimes its bottom so that more signals pass between them for the rhythmic, muscular movements to begin. The softened cervical muscles contract out of the way so that the opening widens. While this is happening, the baby pushes and wriggles into the best position to pass through the birth canal. The mother needs to be free to move around and gently relax into this dance, at this stage more than ever, she needs the belief, faith and trust in her own body's ability.

The second stage then starts with the mother's abdominal muscles pushing the baby along the passage and out into the world.

In a unique way, space is made to accommodate the baby. While the bones in the mother's pelvis expand, those in the baby's head are compressed and massaged as it passes through the birth canal. Gravity s a great help here and it is usually at this stage when a woman wants to be more upright for the surge that follows. Now, however, a quick burst of adrenaline (foetal ejection reflex) is desirable to give the necessary surge of power required to complete the birth. It is an incredible feeling: a mixture of stretching, gushing of water and the speedy sensations of limbs coming out. In a flash it is over, the baby is born.

*"Birth, as experienced by the mother, is the Mount Everest of physical functions in any mammal."*

**Ina May Gaskin**

## What do I need to think about during the birth?

Women have given birth since the dawn of time. Women's bodies are designed for birthing. You are blessed to bring into this world a new being.

Bring calmness and relaxation into your world. Relaxation not only relieves the pain, it allows the body to open up and for the baby to glide into this world. Releasing the breath with each contraction/surge is vital. Using the Alexander technique of "whispered ah's" is the best I know. To do this, you breathe out through the mouth with the tongue touching the bottom teeth and whisper "ah" in a steady, slow stream.

Visualising the waves of the sea worked beautifully for me and for many others. I just imagined the contraction to be like a wave, a surge of energy and I just went with the flow. Allow yourself to be carried on the crest of the wave. The art is to tune into the rhythm and catch them each time.

This is the time to allow your intuition to tap into the deep essence of your being, surrounding yourself in white light.

Some of the thoughts that have helped women in labour:

*I trust, open my heart and believe in my being to
help this baby come joyfully into the world.*

*I am safe, safe, safe. I connect to the countless
millions of women who have given birth before.*

*I send loving energy to the baby inside me
and gently massage it into this world.*

*I am relaxed, relaxed, relaxed. I close my eyes and
allow myself to be swept along in this sea of energy.*

*I allow myself to open up the passageways for this new being.*

Voice any fears as they come up and feel free to make whatever noise
helps, soft deep moans, the lower the better so that it vibrates the lower
part of your body. Trust and let go.

## The vagina seems so small to me. How can a baby possibly pass through?

A concern many women have is how can a baby pass through such a
seemingly, small aperture, the vagina? As Ina May Gaskin points out in
"Guide to Childbirth", the vagina can greatly increase in size, only women
never see it and are not aware of its powers. Men take it for granted that
their sexual organs can greatly increase in size and then become small
again without being damaged. Women's genitals have similar abilities.
After all, women can adapt to any size penis! No measuring has to go on
first to see if it will work or not! How absurd it would be if, before having
a sexual relationship with someone, couples had to go to the doctor to be
measured! So why on earth do we measure the size of the baby's head and
then decide whether it is the right size or not? This is where we come back
to trusting in our bodies' natural processes.

Another important point is engorgement. When a man's penis is erect, the skin has not only become stretched, it has become engorged as well. This happens in women too, only it is not visible, but is noticed by a "tingly" feeling. In birth, just as in sexual foreplay, this engorgement occurs and if a woman's tissues are not well engorged then damage such as tearing is more likely. For some women to increase vaginal engorgement, stimulation of the clitoris can help as the baby emerges.

With this understanding, it can be seen that to artificially cut the vaginal entry to make room for the baby is complete nonsense. This procedure, known as an "episiotomy" has been called "female genital mutilation." Routine episiotomy has no benefits and it can cause pain that can last for weeks. The tissue will never be as was and it can become infected and the pain may prevent the establishment of breastfeeding.

## *How do I know when my labour starts?*

Labour can start in a number of different ways. For example, there can be a "show," which is when the plug of mucus that seals the uterus is passed from the vagina. Or it can start when the forewaters break. These are the initial fluids released before the cervix is fully dilated. Or labour can start when you experience a feeling of 'period like' contractions. Immediately, the best thing to do is to think of going to sleep, staying warm and undisturbed so that the brain can continue making the hormones necessary for your labour to proceed smoothly.

Now imagine that you and your baby are protected by a wonderful white light and say to yourself, "I ask for the courage, the strength and the belief that I can give birth and I trust that all goes well for me and my baby and that this is a joyful experience for us both."

A 'show' is very common and, if not understood, can cause panic. It is, however, a very positive sign, showing that the cervix is nearly ready to dilate.

# What happens if my waters break and I don't feel any contractions?

It is quite common for the bag of waters to rupture without contractions. It is known as premature rupture of the membranes. It is best to go back to bed (use a sanitary towel which you should keep and show to the midwife who can check the colour). Relax, do not switch on the light, close the curtains if it is daylight and allow your brain the time to send the messages round your body. Contractions will soon start.

If a Midwife offers to do a vaginal examination at this point, say no! It would only be to gauge the thickness of the cervix to give her a picture of when the baby might be born. It is not necessary and, what is more, there is a risk of introducing microbes or germs into the vagina and a possible further risk of the newborn baby needing antibiotics after the birth.

Sometimes there is talk of inducing the baby at this stage but, again, it is not necessary and interferes with the birth processes. A randomised Swedish study looked at two groups of women where one group was allowed to continue without interference and the other group was induced. The conclusion was there was no reason to rush to induce.

The only cause for concern is where any leaking fluids are stained dark black, which could be a sign of distress from the baby and results from the baby passing a bowel motion before it is born.

# What happens if I go into labour in an unexpected place such as a car or train?

Don't panic. Allow nature to take its course. Just be sure the place is warm enough so that when the baby is born it can be placed straight onto the mother's chest to allow skin to skin contact. This encourages the final contractions to deliver the placenta, the final part of the birthing process.

One mother had her baby in the car. Her husband simply turned up the heater and left her to it. It turned out to be very straightforward and easy.

If, for some reason, the baby is in a breech position (buttocks or feet first), don't help by pulling as the baby will become stuck. A study of breech births and ambulance calls showed that in cases where the ambulance arrived after the baby was born, the babies were fine; where the ambulance arrived prior to the birth, more babies died or were brain damaged.

## *If I am overdue and it is suggested to rupture my membranes (have my waters broken), what is likely to happen?*

Usually after artificial rupture of the membranes, synthetic oxytocin is likely to be prescribed. This interferes with your body's production of this hormone and the chemical version does not cross the blood brain barrier. Under these circumstances, the body does not make enough of its own hormone and the positive effect of the internally released hormone on the brain, the feeling of euphoria, is lost. It is a lonely experience being induced and it is irreversible. Contractions come very fast and furiously and 90% of women go on to have epidurals as the pain becomes so intense.

There is a small possibility that artificial rupture of the membranes could bring on the very serious condition, placenta abruptio, the separation of placenta from the uterine wall.

When the baby is overdue, or 41 weeks from the last period and coming into the 42nd week, it is important to check daily that the baby is fine. This can be done by combining several methods:

1. Check how many times a day the baby kicks and watch to see if this rate declines or not. Consistent or increasing frequency is a very good sign, a declining rate might indicate a problem.

2. Watch the size of your abdomen: it should increase slightly. If it appears to have shrunk from the previous day, this could be an emergency situation as the fluid surrounding the baby is disappearing.

3. Amnioscopy: this involves a clear tube with a light, the size of a finger, being inserted into the cervix to see the colour of the liquid. If it is beautifully clear, all is well.

4. A urine sample is taken to measure the hormone levels.

5. At this overdue stage, ultrasound scans are very useful to check if a normal amount of liquid is present. This accurate test, unfortunately not often used at this stage, detects immediately if action is needed, including Caesarean section.

## In what position is a baby normally born?

The most common way is headfirst. This is known as a head presentation where the crown presents itself and the head is completely flexed. The baby can be facing to the mother's back, side or tummy. Sometimes the head is not flexed and the face comes first.

All the above are known as eutacic presentations so the baby can be born through the vaginal passage. However, there is one head presentation that makes a natural birth not possible, known as dystocic (a brow presentation). In this very rare situation, a Caesarean section is usually necessary although the 'pelvic press' technique, pioneered by Ina May Gaskin, has been used very successfully.

Occasionally, the baby's head comes out but there is a slight wait for the shoulders to follow; this is known as shoulder distortia. The best thing in this situation is to go into a supported squatting position or onto all fours (the Gaskin manoeuvre) and WAIT. Do not talk; be silent and calm and allow your body's hormones to send the messages and the baby will come in its own good time!

There are times when the baby is not head down but feet down, this is known as a breech position. Most people are told that this situation demands a Caesarean section and that it is incompatible with a home birth. This need not be so. If we go back to understanding the way the body is physiologically designed for birth, there is no reason why a baby cannot be born, vaginally, in a breech position.

In fact, there are many women who have had wonderful birth experiences with their babies born in this way. Someone I know recently had a home birth where she delivered twins, one of whom was in a breech position. It is a good idea to allow the birth process to start naturally. During the first stage of labour, it will be clear whether the vaginal route is possible or not. At least the baby will have the benefit of the natural hormones which are so important. Just bear in mind that the principles of privacy, silence, low lighting, warmth and the comfort of the mother - with no observers - still apply.

In a breech birth, the pattern of labour is slightly different. It is not so fast at the beginning: the head is not pushing down but the feet are, so there is less contact and weight. But as soon as the buttocks give the last touch to the cervix, complete dilation will occur.

## As the father, what should I do at the birth?

Ideally the father's role is to be the protector and, as long as you understand the basic physiological (how the body operates) needs of a woman in labour, you are in a good position to help.

Don't feel obliged to be constantly present, actively doing things, or asking questions. It is much more important that you see to the needs of others at this time, such as making sure there is food for everyone or filling the birthing pool, leave the mother to do her job. If she sees you watching her, your presence will actively slow the release of the important hormones that are being made by her brain and are telling her body what to do.

Most men are relieved by this direction. However, understanding the reasons will avoid any feelings of being left out.

# What is a doula?

A doula is a female companion, almost like a mother/grandmother figure who attends the birth. Unfortunately in this day and age, midwives have to follow so much paperwork and bureaucracy that, on occasions, they are unable to be "the quiet calm presence of a wise woman waiting in the wings who, by her very presence, is enough to reassure the labouring mother" (Michel Odent). Odent's Paramanadoulas (Greek for slave to the mother) help before the birth to explain the basic needs of a woman in labour to reduce the stimulation of the logical thinking brain so that the archaic brain structures become active, so vital for labour. At the birth such a doula will do everything possible to help the mother by bringing silence, darkness, privacy and calmness to the arena as well as assisting the midwife in anyway she can.

# Will I feel awkward or embarrassed during labour?

In my own independent research, one of the fears that came up time and time again was the concern of bodily functions during labour. It is true that the bowels empty but usually this happens early on in labour when it is still quite easy to go to the loo. If anything does happen later on, midwives are trained to deal with the situation and would know how to remove it straight away. In most cases, no one would even notice and it would only be a very small amount. It is also true that women make very strange noises but I can reassure you that when it comes to it, nothing is embarrassing. We are not used to anyone dealing with our private parts, but at the birth everything is so extraordinary that these fears that may seem important now simply do not arise, they just melt away!

# Are there tips to help during the birth?

Encouraging the body to relax is of prime importance. Laughter is excellent, especially, a good belly laugh. Ina May Gaskin, one of the leading midwives of our time, tells some wonderful stories where, through observation of hundreds of births, she has learned some great tips. Shaking the thighs is one of them. She has found that if the thigh muscles are tense then so are the pelvic floor muscles. By gently and rhythmically shaking the thighs from side to side during a contraction or two helps the woman to relax and let go! Equally she has observed that relaxing the jaw helps. Women whose mouths and throats are opened and relaxed during labour and birth rarely need stitches due to a tear or need cutting (episiotomy).

She gives a practical tip for people who are constipated and have difficulty evacuating - open your mouth and relax your jaw!

Another suggestion is to suggest to pregnant women that they imagine themselves to be a large mammal when they are in labour. Imagine being a large ape and making monkey noises can help women to find the primate in them and connect to the successful births in this world!

# What are the methods of induction?

The medical way is to give medication (prostaglandins) which prepare the cervix so that it becomes soft and flat ready to dilate. In some cases a gel can be used and in other cases synthetic oxytocin via a drip can be used.

The physical method is called "sweeping the membranes." This is when a midwife or obstetrician separates the membranes from the cervix, it is thought to stimulate the release of prostaglandins.

Acupuncture and Reflexology sessions are treatments that seem to be effective in stimulating labour.

An old fashioned method is to drink castor oil, this is not advisable and leads to diarrhoea.

It is very important to understand that if the baby is ready to come, it is also producing its own hormones thus stimulating the mother's own production. These hormones are chemical messengers that help cells to communicate with each other. Encouraging the mother to relax and trust in her own body's capabilities is the best advice. If, however, the baby is not ready then any method of induction interferes with the natural physiological processes. Make sure you are informed as to your choices at this stage.

## How do I increase my chances of having an un-medicated labour and birth in hospital?

Visit the hospital or birthing centre first. Most likely, you will be visiting the hospital anyway for your antenatal check-ups; ask where the birthing room or rooms are situated and request a tour. It is very important to familiarise yourself first. Check out if there is a birthing pool and where the nearest shower is located. Having a shower during labour can be a wonderful way of shutting down the thinking brain and having the privacy that you need. Spraying water onto the nipples will stimulate oxytocin release and help labour to progress.

Take an aroma burner and burn some essential oils such as tea tree (antiseptic) and lavender (calming). It may not be possible to burn candles as they can be a fire hazard but find out and take some night-lights, which are much safer, or an electrically operated aroma burner.

There is usually a physio ball and/or a bean bag to use during labour.

Drink plenty of water. Oxygenated water can be a real boon, add some liquid minerals and you have an excellent drink. Going to the loo also helps to relax the pelvic muscles.

Take a comfortable dressing gown, robe, nightshirt, or big T-shirt.

Consider hiring a Doula. Studies show that having one cuts the odds in half of having an unwanted Caesarean. It also halves the odds of having a forceps or vacuum-extraction delivery, as well as shortening labour by greatly reducing stress, pain and anxiety.

## *Tell me about Caesarean section.*

This is when the baby is cut out of the mother's body with the use of anaesthetic medication. A four-inch horizontal incision is made just above the pubic bone. This can be a wonderful rescue operation when birth through the vaginal canal is not possible.

Compared with vaginal birth, Caesarean section carries increased risks of death and permanent injury. It takes a physical and emotional toll and increases the incidence of babies born in poor condition with breathing problems, jaundice and admission to special-care units. Accidental surgical injury to the mother's bowel, bladder, uterus, or uterine blood vessels occurs in some cases and may necessitate a blood transfusion due to excessive blood loss. Risk of infection, blood clots to the legs and even septicaemia (blood poisoning) are possibilities.

Beginning motherhood while recovering from major surgery is not easy, plus the natural hormones have not been allowed to pass between mother and baby. As a result depression is more likely with difficulties forming an attachment to the baby.

Dispelling some myths:

- Caesarean section does not prevent urinary incontinence, faecal incontinence and sexual dysfunction.

- You do not regain your figure so quickly.

- Caesarean is more likely to cause injury to the vagina, pelvic floor and the perineum (area between the vagina and the anus) than a natural vaginal birth. These injuries nearly always arise from episiotomies (cutting the vaginal opening to enlarge it) and forceps and vontuse procedures.

- If you had a Caesarean before, you do not have to have one again (VBAC Vaginal Birth after Caesarean).

- Women are twice as likely to suffer a stillbirth next time and on average it is four times harder for a woman to become pregnant again. The reasons for reduced fertility probably involve several factors including trauma of the operation, scar tissue in the womb and infections as well as the psychological effect on the mother.

In fact, passing through the vaginal passageway does not hurt or damage the baby. On the contrary, it receives enormous benefits: its head is massaged, thus stimulating its brain and spinal cord. It also receives the protective bacteria from its mother's vaginal secretions, which is of vital importance. A baby is born sterile. Having never been exposed to germs externally it is suddenly exposed to countless millions of these microbes, so it is far better that the first germs it does come into contact with are those from its own mother (inbuilt immunity in the womb). This is yet another example of nature's blueprint for survival.

## *Is my milk different if I have a Caesarean section compared to an uninterrupted vaginal birth?*

Yes! Mother's milk and colostrum (secretion which comes through the breast in the first few days before the milk comes through) both contain opiates which cause the baby to crave its mother's milk, make the baby feel good and help the mother/baby bond. Studies in Italy have measured the amount of beta-endorphins in milk (morphine like hormones) and found that there were significant amounts in the milk after an unmedicated vaginal birth as opposed to a Caesarean section.

# My first baby was born by Caesarean section. Is it still possible to have a vaginal birth?

Definitely yes! This is commonly known as VBAC (vaginal birth after Caesarean section). Women are sometimes told that they will rupture after a previous Caesarean, there is a risk but only around 0.5%. However, if the labour is induced, either physically or medically, then uterine rupture increases 10 fold. So, if offered an induction the next time round after having had a C- section, you have the right to allow your body to go into labour naturally. If you understand how important it is to encourage the body's production of key hormones, including oxytocin and all that it entails, you will significantly increase your success rate.

# If, after everything, I have to have an epidural, what can I expect?

The painkilling medication is given by injecting anaesthetic into the lower back just outside the spinal cord through a fine plastic tube. This is left in place so that the medication can be added if the anaesthetic wears off. For the tube to be inserted, the pregnant woman must curl forward to increase the space between the bones of the spine. This is a very uncomfortable position when the baby is in the way! The epidural numbs and weakens the lower part of the body.

Epidurals do have side effects:

- There can be a dramatic drop in blood pressure which can affect both the mother's and the baby's heart rate. Another interference then occurs through the addition of an intravenous infusion (a drip) to help normalise the blood pressure.

- 1 in 5 women have a fever which means the baby will need a needle jab on arrival into the world with the crucial "critical hour" bonding with its mother being broken.

- In approximately 2% of epidurals, accidental lumbar punctures occur, which means that the needle went in too far and punctured the spinal cord membrane. As a result, no epidural can then be given and the mother ends up with a severe headache that lasts for days or even weeks.

- Some women react to the medication and develop severe itching all over their bodies.

- Epidurals don't always work. Some women do not have any relief. Some receive only partial relief meaning they feel the contractions in one patch or on one side. There is simply nothing to be done but to grin and bear it. The body will not be making its own painkillers or its "feel good" hormones either.

- In rare cases, 1 in 1000 epidurals can result in permanent paralysis to the woman or even death.

- Some women feel totally separated from the whole process. Some have said they even feel "like a piece of meat" as they are wheeled on to the trolley after delivery. One woman I interviewed said she was put onto a trolley and left alone in the room and realised that her leg was slipping off and she could do nothing to stop herself falling off!

- Women, who initially opt for an epidural, never intend to have a forceps or vontuse (vacuum) extraction and are disappointed when it has to happen.

- There can be some unpleasant after effects such as infection from the needle puncture and injury or muscular strain from poor positioning during birth. A woman cannot feel if her body is in an awkward position.

- Afterwards the baby may not establish breastfeeding easily. The baby can be dopey with the medication, or it may have the critical bonding time with its mother disturbed.

Do not feel under any pressure whatsoever to have an epidural. You have the right to opt for a natural birth. If, however, you have to have one make sure you are aware of the dangers, have people around who you can trust and have an understanding of the "critical hour" for bonding time so that you can give your baby as much emotional security as it arrives into this world.

## *Having decided to have a homebirth, are there any situations when I should abandon the plan and go to hospital?*

Yes. Your midwife/health professional will know about these rare occasions when something happens unexpectedly. The following five situations have to be handled in a hospital.

- If the contractions are coming every 5 minutes with each lasting for only 1 minute and it has been going on for more than one hour, then go to hospital. Continued contractions of this nature could cause restricted blood flow to the baby.

- There is also Placenta Abruption. The placenta can separate from the uterine wall, either partially or completely, during labour before the birth of the baby. This usually occurs with awful and continuous abdominal pain, bleeding may or may not happen. This is when a scan can show very quickly what is going on, to assess whether an immediate operation is needed or not. More often than not, there is no known cause for this but it could be as result of serious trauma such as a car accident during pregnancy.

- Another case is Placenta Praevia. In this instance, the placenta covers the cervix and blocks the way for the baby to be delivered through the birth canal. A scan at this stage is extremely useful.

- As mentioned earlier, Brow Presentation is when the forehead comes first and this is generally incompatible with the vaginal route.

- The one single serious emergency of which to be aware is Cord Prolapse. However, this is very rare and affects only 2 out of every 15,000 births. It occurs when the umbilical cord can be seen coming out of the vulva before the baby is born. If you are not already in hospital then go there as quickly as possible. Whoever is helping you should telephone in advance, or on the way, so that a medical team will be ready for an emergency caesarean section. The baby's head could well be compressing the cord, cutting off the blood supply from the placenta.

All the above cases are safely managed in a hospital environment, so there is one thought that should dominate: BE CALM. It is vital for the expectant mother not to be anxious in any way so as to prevent any further distress or complications. All professionals know how to deal with any of these unlikely situations and if you are reading this before giving birth, know that whatever position a baby is in, having an active birth will enable your body and your baby to find the right position when it comes to the birth itself. Then the above complications rarely happen. "Trust and let go" is the powerful thought that should dominate your mind.

## How did the use of birthing pools start?

Michel Odent, a well known obstetrician and a true pioneer in understanding the birth processes, looked for a way of reducing adrenaline levels in difficult labours after all the basic considerations had been addressed: warmth, hunger, privacy, soft lighting and peace and quiet. This includes the removal of anyone who was stressed and releasing adrenaline such as the father, the midwife, or the doctor.

Odent wondered if water would help the labour to progress in such a way that would reduce the need for painkilling medication. So in the 1970's in a French state hospital in Pithiviers, he began immersing women in water heated to body temperature (no hotter) and the short term results were reduction in pain, lowered stress levels and more oxytocin release, resulting in more effective contractions. The long term result was the redistribution of blood, more to the chest than to the extremities. The heart is sensitive to blood volume and itself releases a hormone which modulates the posterior lobe of the pituitary gland helping the birth process; this takes 1 ½ to 2 hours.

He also found that anticipating the bath and the noise of the water filling up the pool itself was often enough for dilation of the cervix to progress so much so that some babies were born on the floor by the pool even before the pool was ready. His pharmacy bill dropped! So he set up an aquatic birthing room, which was painted blue and decorated with dolphins. From 1970 to 1983, 1000 women used the pool with great success.

It was written up in the Lancet (a medical journal) in 1983 stating that immersion in water at body temperature was an effective and cheap way of reducing drugs in labour and at the same time he warned colleagues that it was bound to happen that a baby **MAY BE** born in water (not that it **SHOULD** be born in water). This attracted a lot of publicity. Then in August 1999, the British Medical Journal (BMJ) published a large study investigating babies being born in water and stated that very few deaths occurred. This study changed the focus to having babies born in water rather than the objective of assisting a difficult labour and reducing the need for painkillers and intervention.

## *Do all hospitals have birthing pools?*

Yes. In the **UK** all **NHS** hospitals that have birthing centres have a birthing pool. Whatever country you are in, find out if this is so and, if not, look for the nearest bathroom facilities where there is running water. A shower can be a great place too. (See recommendations for using a birthing pool).

# *If I am planning a home birth should I rent a birthing pool?*

It is a good idea to rent one, water is a wonderfully relaxing medium. It is really helpful when, in the unlikely event, labour does not progress easily, you, then have the option to immerse yourself in water heated, to body temperature. Just by hearing the sound of water or being near it, can have a miraculous effect. But once in the water, do not stay there for longer than 1 ½ hours, otherwise you can become too tired and the whole process slow down even to a stop.

This is what happened to me, but I did not know this then and as a result, I was exhausted when the baby was born. I should have come out of the water and perhaps gone back later. I also had the water too hot.

# *What are the recommendations for using a birthing pool?*

These are the specific guidelines as recommended by Odent who pioneered the use of water in hospital for difficult birth situations so as to avoid using medication, women and babies shall be eternally grateful to him for this wonderful idea:

1. Don't use the pool too soon, ideally not until the mother's cervix has reached five centimetres dilation. If the mother is impatient to go in, rather early on in the labour, then a shower is most helpful. Directing a jet of water onto the nipples stimulates the release of oxytocin, the hormone needed to help the labour progress! A shower is also a private place and again privacy helps oxytocin production.

2. The birthing pool must be the right temperature 37°C (97°F) or body temperature. If it is too hot, it increases not only the mother's temperature but the unborn baby's temperature too. As the baby's temperature is normally 1 degree higher than the mother's, it uses more oxygen when hot so this can cause foetal distress.

3. Do not plan a birth under water – a mother's body may tell her it is time to come but her mind will insist that she stays in!. Often coming out just before the baby is born stimulates a burst of adrenaline (foetal ejection reflex) now needed for the final push. Staying in the pool for too long can slow down the delivery and exhaust the mother. There are wonderful stories about water birth but there are many more out of the water!

## If, after having been in the pool for 1½ hours labour is not progressing what does it mean?

Check the following criteria have been addressed that allows the mother's instinctive primal brain to work properly:

- no one is watching, videoing, photographing or questioning the mother and

- all her basic considerations such as warmth, hunger, soft lighting and privacy have been addressed

- ensure there is no one around who are themselves stressed and releasing adrenaline as this can affect the woman giving birth very seriously

- the birthing pool was used correctly

- if full dilation has not occurred, then a non-emergency Caesarean section is likely.

## Is it a good idea to plan an underwater birth?

No. A woman whose sole focus is on having her baby delivered in water might risk being a prisoner of her own project.

## My waters have broken. Can I still go into the pool?

Yes. Hard data from a Swedish study supports this.

# *Conclusion*

Sometimes it is helpful to remember that giving birth has been done by countless trillions of women down through the ages from even before Biblical times. Our genetic blueprint carries each one of us through this experience and this extraordinary process. What we are seeking to do is to not only give ourselves the best possible chance but to give our babies the best experience too with a gentle welcome full of joy and love. At the end of the day, if the birth does not work out in the way that you had perhaps hoped for, it doesn't matter. What matters is that both you and your baby are safe. The most important thing is you attempted the kind of birth you believe to be the best. You don't want to look back on the experience and say, "I wish I'd had the courage or confidence to try."

Sometime ago I was consulted by a client during her second pregnancy. Then, as her Doula I was present at the birth and, some weeks later we spent time together and talked through her experience. This is her story:

She woke at 3 a.m. just like the last time. She heaved herself out of bed and went to the loo. There seemed to be some blood on the paper. Was this what is called a show? She immediately looked this up in the book, which was on her bedside. "…could happen up to two days before the baby was born." So she went back to bed and slept for the rest of the night.

In the morning, she woke her husband, John, with the same words as before - "I think something is happening." He rolled over and went back to sleep! This was best thing he could have done as it showed her that he was totally relaxed which made her feel the same. As this was her second pregnancy, she was more familiar with the period like contractions. With John unresponsive, she woke her sister, Sam, who was staying with her. As she went downstairs, she felt glad of the movement and decided to call her mother who was one and a half hours away. After that excitement, she decided to go back to bed. After all it was still dark outside and it had taken a few hours the last time. She slept for a while and when the contractions became stronger and it was impossible to lie in bed, she suddenly realised that she hadn't even packed a bag! After all, her due date was not for 10 days. So quietly, she packed a couple of large shirts (easy for feeding), a nursing bra, a wash bag, minerals and vitamins, linseed, water, essential oils, candles, arnica and some baby clothes.

Then she had breakfast. She knew from last time that she wouldn't be interested in eating later on so she needed good, slow releasing fuel. She ate some homemade, soaked muesli with grated apple, almonds and sunflower seeds. However, her bowels moved twice – a good sign as it shows that the birthing process is really underway. Then her three year old, Angie, woke up and she managed to give her breakfast before she had to start rocking and breathing through the contractions, reminding herself to let go and relax. It was so much worse if she tensed up.

Her husband timed the contractions and they were coming every ten minutes. Then she had one 7 minutes later and the next 5 minutes later. Things were hotting up! She decided it was time to telephone the hospital. It was now 7 a.m.

It was time, now, to go to the hospital. The contractions were very strong and she couldn't possibly sit in the front of the car, so she climbed into the back on all fours and travelled like that for the whole journey. Just as well as suddenly there was a gush of water, her waters broke followed by three intense contractions. Even in her semi-conscious state she was aware that the car was moving very fast!

As she arrived at the hospital entrance she had one very intense contraction and remembers hanging on to the railing and rocking and moaning through it. She was taken straight to the delivery room.

The midwife managed to assess her in an upright position and said she was six centimetres dilated. She continued to work through the contractions in a rhythmical rocking motion. Someone asked her if she wanted to go into the bath and she remembered how the warm water had eased the pain last time so before it was even full she was in on all fours!. As long as she could move, the pain was very manageable.

This helped for a while and then the midwife said it was time to "get out." So somehow she did. She dived straight into a beanbag, she was now kneeling on the floor in a sort of upright position, face into the beanbag.

Now she used her mind. "Tranquillity" was the refrain she kept repeating and she started to visualise the sea and rolling waves. She just imagined that she was part of this movement with little lulls in-between. She kept telling herself to let go, relax and open up. She was also thinking of her body's physical changes and the baby coming out. She moaned and clenched her fingers into the beanbag material. She wanted to make holes in it but it was a strong rubber material and too tough!

Suddenly she was pulled out of my inner world by the midwife who wanted to put on the foetal heart monitor. She tensed through the next contraction only to realise that she tightened up and the contractions became more painful. So she moaned gently and felt her body opening up. She was slightly put off when the midwife said to start panting, but she ignored it and went on with the whispered "ah's."

She was aware of an enormous stretching feeling, the baby was coming. She felt as if she couldn't possibly stretch anymore and knew the baby was there, but it went back again. Another push and out came the baby's head. She asked, "Is it out?" And they said "Yes!" But she still did not have the relief that she was expecting so she knew it was just the head and pushed again. This time there was a gush and out came the baby!

She felt instant relief and moaned into the cushion. "Yehudi was marvellous," she said "he was on all fours behind me!" Then she was told to reach through her legs and pick up her baby. She saw that it was a boy with hardly any hair! No one had told her, they just waited for her to see for herself. She couldn't believe it! How absolutely wonderful! One more push and the placenta came out. This didn't hurt at all. She was absolutely fine. No tearing, no stitches.

She put her new baby straight to her breast and he started to root around and suckle in a newborn manner.

She lay back contentedly. She had done it again! She was tired but euphoric at experiencing feelings that were beyond the realms of words and even of this world.

Eventually, she stood up and walked out of the delivery room. Not the most elegant of walks of course, more like a waddle! The next day she overheard the cleaners saying to each other "Do you know, she even walked out of the delivery room!"

Her general impression of this second natural delivery was how much quicker and easier it was compared to her first. She was not even expecting this baby to arrive until the following week! Her recollections of the next few weeks were how easy this new baby was. He seemed calm and slept well, breastfeeding seemed to fall into place and so began her life with a new born and a toddler.

Now we come to the next step, the "Critical Hour," which makes a huge difference to establishing the maternal/baby bond and all its implications.

# Step 5 - The Critical Hour After Birth

So much discussion and information surrounds birth itself that this Critical Hour immediately afterwards is often completely overlooked or forgotten. The focus is on the birth and the safe delivery of the baby. There is general feeling of the job is done with a rush to tidy up, cut the cord, deliver the placenta and wash the baby. Imagine you are a new born baby, arriving from a warm, safe, watery cocoon to the outside world. Wouldn't you want a joyful welcome? Wouldn't you want to snuggle into a safe, warm place, to find a familiar smell or voice? Who better than the mother who has been carrying you for the past nine months? Who, as she reaches down for you, puts you onto her naked breast with the lovely warmth and comfort of skin to skin contact and then, as both of you look into each other's eyes, linking your hearts and brains, you fall in love. What better reception could you have?

If a baby is received into the world like this, science and psychology show us that this is what happens. If a woman gives birth in the way her body was designed and the hormones and chemical messages are allowed to function as nature intended, then this incredible bonding process occurs. Science has shown that the right brain of both mother and baby synchronise with each other in an "infant-leads, mother-follows sequence." Then as the baby reaches up to its mother's breast, its mouth opens and latches onto her nipple and starts sucking.

The importance of this interaction cannot be underestimated. In their book The Secret Life of the Unborn Child, Thomas Verny and John Kelly, leading authorities on the effect of the unborn baby's and infant's environment said as long ago as 1981 "Study after study has shown that women who bond with their babies become better mothers and their babies almost always are physically healthier, emotionally more stable and intellectually more acute than infants separated from their mothers right after birth"

If you give birth in a hospital, make sure to notify your doctor or midwife in advance of your desire to keep the baby with you immediately after the birth, not to be disturbed and not to let any routine procedures happen such as washing, weighing, measuring, wiping the baby's eyes or cutting the umbilical cord (this should not happen until the placenta is delivered). You can explain that you would like the vernix, the baby's protective coating, to be left on the skin. Sometimes a tube is put into the baby's mouth or its nose to suck out any fluids. This again does not have to be done with every birth.

## *What is the importance of these hormones that are made in this Critical Hour?*

If these hormones are not allowed to be produced and the bonding does not occur properly, there is the potential of spoiling the child's capacity to love not only itself, but others too. In other words, lack of these hormones would increase the potential for impairing the baby's future relationships. Isn't this extraordinary? If you find some of this hard to believe, then take a look at the research Primal Health Research Editorial (Winter 1994, Vol. 2, No. 3) entitled "Preventing Violence or Developing the Capacity to Love."

# What happens immediately after the baby is born?

The third stage of the birth process is expelling the placenta. The womb continues to contract helping the placenta to come away from its wall and, as this happens, usually fifteen to twenty minutes after the birth, dark red blood is passed. Finally after a few more contractions, the placenta is expelled; this is known as the "afterbirth."

Now comes the newborn period sometimes known as the fourth stage of labour. This includes the first six weeks that follow childbirth. During this time breastfeeding is established, so the best thing for your baby is to be put straight to the mother's breast, skin to skin, even before cutting the umbilical cord. Breastfeeding is so instinctive in humans that it is almost a guarantee for the baby to suckle within the first hour. It is very important that the mother is not disturbed in anyway and that the natural contractions continue for the placenta to be expelled of its own accord. The cord should not be cut until this occurs.

The body starts preparing for the production of milk early on in the pregnancy. In fact, at 19 weeks into the pregnancy, lactose can be detected in the urine of a pregnant woman. The main hormones involved with milk production are oxytocin, prolactin and prostaglandins. Studies show that natural painkillers (beta endorphins) are released, which subsequently releases prolactin. Oxytocin is pulsed into the blood stream during labour and the more effectively it is pulsed into the blood stream, the quicker the milk will flow.

To establish breastfeeding successfully, we should not interfere with the birth processes. Caesarean sections prevent the body from making these necessary hormones. In Countries where Caesarian rates are high, there are very active politics for promoting breastfeeding and some countries even suggest substances to help milk secretion. People are unaware of the link between birth as nature intended and the ability to successfully breastfeed.

# What to do

Put the baby straight to the breast. Babies who suckle in this first hour are unlikely to have jaundice. Allow the mother and baby time to rest and recover from the physical exertion that has just occurred. Keep the room warm and cover them loosely with a sheet or blanket, allowing the baby to lie naked at its mother's breast.

- Do not cut the cord until the placenta is expelled.

- Do not disturb the mother and baby in any way.

- Allow the placenta to be expelled in its own time.

## *I have heard that you can haemorrhage after giving birth.*

According to research, postpartum haemorrhages (bleeding after the baby is born) are almost always related to inappropriate interference. What this means is that a few basic concepts need to be understood. Just as the baby is about to be born, there is an automatic reflex that occurs called the "foetal ejection reflex." This is a short series of contractions that push the baby out. This can only occur if the mother is producing the right hormones and, for this to happen, she must be in an environment of calm where everyone has low levels of adrenaline.

The mother usually goes to an upright position at the moment of birth. As soon as the baby is born, warm the room (plan in advance for extra heaters or if in hospital use an overhead heater). Do not disturb the mother in any way. She must not be spoken to or interfered with whatsoever. She needs be to in state of semi-consciousness, almost a sleep state, so that her brain continues to make the hormones necessary to let the final stage of labour proceed - the separation of the placenta from her womb and then the last few contractions to expel it.

Active management during the third stage of labour, i.e. if it is managed medically, is something you absolutely do not want! This results in all the natural mechanisms shutting down and there is far greater risk of excessive bleeding which can even lead to a blood transfusion. Active management also interferes with your bonding and special time with your baby.

## *Is there any way of preventing this?*

Yes. An easy delivery of the placenta with moderate blood loss can only occur if a surge of oxytocin has been released. It is well known that oxytocin release is highly dependent on environmental factors and can be inhibited by adrenaline. Postpartum haemorrhages are associated with high levels of adrenaline. Make sure the following occurs to avoid the hazards:

- Warm the room with heating lamps or a transportable heater (use extension cable if needed).

- Nobody should be around the mother and baby other than a motherly, silent and low-profile midwife sitting and knitting in a corner. Knitting or a similar repetitive task helps the midwife to keep her own level of adrenaline as low as possible.

- No observation by anyone.

- Silence, no talking, TV, radio or telephone.

- Dimmed lights with curtains or blinds closed tightly.

- Do not touch mother or baby for one hour following the birth.

If the placenta has not been delivered after one hour has passed, check to see if the placenta has separated from the uterus. With the mother on her back, press the abdominal wall with the fingertips just above the pubic bone. If the cord does not move, it means that the placenta is separated. (For further research, consult Primal Health Research, Autumn 2004, Vol. 12, No.2).

# What is best to eat and drink in this Critical Hour?

Oxygenated water and colloidal minerals can still be drunk. Thirst should be quenched with water, not sweet, sugary drinks. Often well-meaning members of the family and friends bring in champagne and alcohol. Avoid this at all costs as it ends up going into the baby and can cause colic. This is a quiet time of rest and bonding. There is usually no desire for food.

# Tell me about the newborn period sometimes known as the fourth stage of labour, including the first six weeks that follow childbirth?

If you have had your baby without any medical intervention, you will find your body recovers extremely quickly after the birth. You may feel tired but then who wouldn't after a marathon? Breastfeeding stimulates the uterus to continue contracting (very mild) so that you regain your figure very quickly. With gentle stomach exercises, starting with a few pelvic floor squeezes daily (imagine squeezing a pencil), your stomach will be toned and go back to its shape, too. If however, you have had an epidural and intravenous lines put into your veins, you may suffer long-term from backache and your body may hurt for a while. It is rather a paradox that although orthodox medicine's main criteria is to relieve childbirth pain, it actually ends up giving real, hurtful pain afterwards with no euphoria whatsoever.

# *Conclusion*

This Critical Hour is a time of great spiritual connection. The joy and wonder of the arrival of a new human being is so incredible that for most women, they are coasting in a different reality. The joy is immense although there may be feelings of physical exhaustion. One of the best kept secrets is that birth can be ecstatic and strengthening giving inner power and wisdom. If it is not it has many implications. The following is taken from the practice:

Keith, a man in his mid forties, came to me in desperation. His whole world had been turned upside down. His wife of nearly 10 years had walked out on him with their two children Adam and Susan, aged 8 and 6, because he said, "She couldn't stand living any longer with someone so emotionally cold and depressing." Keith was experiencing a number of different health problems: he had a chronic low back problem (which sometimes left him crippled with such pain forcing bed rest), asthma, disturbed sleeping patterns, constipation and digestive disturbances. He had never been to a holistic practitioner of any description, only to his doctor.

As I went through his case history, he answered with an expressionless and monotonous voice and never once looked at me. I couldn't seem to connect to him emotionally, but I worked hard at trying to engage him and having answers to the questions, otherwise the consultation was going nowhere. As I continued with the case history we came to the subject of how he was born. Did he know?

He told me that his mother had had an unexpected pregnancy and did not want "the child" (he said this in a detached way using the third party). She became very depressed after the birth and struggled to look after him. He never even knew his father. Eventually she met and married someone else and life became easier. At school, Keith had been a loner, he never really had any friends and in fact he was bullied at school. He had an obsession with making match stick models and immersed himself in numbers, excelling in mathematics. Now he was a Government analyst.

Finally Keith said that he had been diagnosed with Asperger's syndrome. This explained everything, in fact I had come to this conclusion and wondered if he knew about it. People who have this are emotionally inept, they can't understand emotion or empathise with others. It makes social situations almost impossible and they always have strange eye contact, either none at all or a staring manner. Research shows that lack of bonding and attachment to the mother plays a significant role in causing this cold, socially unacceptable behaviour. With all that we have read about birth and the importance of allowing the 'love hormone,' oxytocin, to flow, this story demonstrates what the outcome can be.

*"During pregnancy, as your body undertakes the physical formation of a fetus, your mind undertakes the formation of an idea of the mother you might become. ..... In a sense, there are three pregnancies going on simultaneously: the physical fetus growing in your womb, the motherhood mindset developing in your psyche, and the imagined baby taking shape in your mind."*

**Stern, Bruschweiler-Stern and Freeland**
Authors of *The Birth of a Mother*

# Step 6 - Early Motherhood

Becoming a mother is a wonderful but demanding role, never more so than in the first few weeks. This final step gives tips and advice of some of the most common concerns at this stage. This is also a very physically demanding time and requires plenty of energy. It is, however, the most wonderful time and it is good to remember that on some days everything goes smoothly and on others it does not. So what? Roll on to the next one! Life is a bit like juggling balls, sometimes they are all up in the air and sometimes they are all on the floor in a heap. The main thing is to keep a sense of humour and do your best to laugh. Before you can blink your baby will be smiling, one of the greatest joys in life.

## *My baby, only a few hours old, has a high temperature. Does she/he need antibiotics?*

It is important to remember that if a mother has had an epidural the thermo-regulation of her temperature is paralysed and so the baby may have a higher temperature anyway. Always ask for the swab results before antibiotics are given. Remember also that breastfeeding and the first liquid from the mother (colostrum) helps the immune system, the system which fights illness.

# *My body looks so strange. Will I ever look like I did before I was pregnant?*

It can be rather a surprise to look at oneself after the baby has been born because everything does not just go back into shape straight away. The muscles and ligaments have all been stretched, but they DO all go back and there is no reason why you should not regain your figure. Breastfeeding speeds this process, as every time the baby suckles, this action stimulates the muscles of the womb to contract which means your tummy goes flatter. It is very important to do gentle pelvic floor exercises. It is customary to have a six-week check up with your doctor or health professional and then you can start to do more intensive stomach exercises.

All the effort that you have put into yourself before and during the pregnancy will pay off and you will be surprised how soon you will be back in shape. So when you have your first shower or bath and look at a very flabby tummy, do not be disturbed. Take comfort from the animal kingdom: after the mother gives birth, she returns to normal.

For those of you who have had pets who have had babies, you will know so well and so it is with us providing we have followed the Wellness Action Plan. If this is not the case, start it now. It is never too late. If given the right messages, the body always heals and repairs itself.

# *When do I start exercising?*

You can start exercising when the body feels ready, but it is not wise to go into a full stretch routine or to run a marathon as there is a danger of overstretching and injury as the hormone, relaxin, stays in your system for up to sixteen weeks after birth. It is very important to start gentle pelvic floor exercises a few days after the birth. The simple way to locate these muscles is by stopping the urine flow midstream, hold for a second and then resume. However don't continue to repeat this as it could irritate the water works and cause infection. Now that you have located these muscles and now recognise the feeling, you can repeat this as often as possible during the day. Make it a habit to do a few repetitions when brushing your teeth or sitting feeding your baby.

## *What breastfeeding tips do you have?*

Keep your baby near to you especially at the beginning. This contact is essential for bonding and it allows you to know when the baby needs feeding. This is especially so at night: if you have the baby near you, you can easily lift him or her for feeding without either of you being disturbed too much - you literally feed in your sleep. It is very important not to put the lights on or to play and talk, so that the baby starts to understand the difference between day and night.

To avoid most of the common problems that occur in the first few weeks such as sore nipples, engorgement (when the breast becomes very hard) and mastitis (see question below), make sure the baby is attached to the breast properly with the nipple fully in the mouth and is put to the breast often enough. With breastfeeding, it is useful to ask your midwife, or someone who has had experience, for help with positioning, technique and posture. For example, when taking the baby off the breast (perhaps fallen asleep), insert your little finger into the corner of the baby's mouth so that you don't drag the mouth off your nipple.

A first time mother needs help with her own body posture while feeding to avoid building up muscular tension, cushions and pillows are very helpful. The key is to relax and not hurry, don't let your mind flip backwards or forwards, thinking of things that should have been or need to be done. Enjoy the present moment, it is very special.

Each time you sit down to feed, have a muslin cloth handy and a glass of water. The cloth is for your shoulder to make it nice and soft for the baby's face or to catch any milk that comes out when winding your baby. The water is for you, the mother. It is crucial to drink 3 – 4 litres/5-7 pints a day (3 for the mother and 1 for the baby). I once asked a herdsman what difference it made to cow's milk production if the water supply was cut off. Without any hesitation, he said there was an immediate drop in milk volume and even a loss of as little as 24 hours could take a week for supplies to return to normal! Difficulty with breastfeeding is usually due to the mother's lack of water or insufficient rest. Follow the Wellness Action Plan guidelines in step one.

Breast milk contains all the food and water your baby needs for the first six months. Giving other food or drink could be harmful and may also make the baby less interested in breastfeeding. The sucking action plays a valuable part in a baby's physical and emotional development. Sometimes there is a bit of work required to make the milk flow and this is nature's design. A hungry baby will suck more frequently to increase the supply and this is the miraculous thing about breastfeeding. You, the mother, don't need to think about how much milk is being consumed, just trust nature to do it for you.

The beauty of breastfeeding is that you can be out and about with your baby and know that there is a constant supply of food at all times. Wear clothes that open easily or are specially designed for feeding, so that when you are out and breastfeeding, no breast shows. It really can be a very discreet process. I found a sling to be wonderful, no one even knew when I was feeding.

If the breast becomes hard, it is engorged. Putting a cabbage leaf inside the nursing bra is an old trick and it works! I know this from both my personal and from others' experiences, too.

There are some wonderful organizations which support breastfeeding mothers – La Leche League, an international organization, The National Childbirth Trust (NCT) in the UK and the UNICEF UK Baby Friendly Initiative.

# What is mastitis? What can you do to prevent it and what can be done when you have it?

Mastitis is a blocked milk duct. This causes a lump which can become red and painful due to bacterial infection. To avoid it, make sure that each time you feed your baby, one breast is emptied completely before you swap sides. Don't start each feed on the same breast, as a hungry baby will suck harder initially.

The nipple, like a showerhead, has lots of little holes and sometimes, one or two become blocked. By gently massaging the breast in the direction of the nipple, a mother can free the flow. A hot bath also helps increase the circulation, as do alternating hot and cold flannels compressed on the breast. Also, make sure you encourage the baby to suck every time on the breast that is causing concern, as this is the best way to overcome the problem.

Always have the homeopathic remedy, phytolacca to hand. It works miracles!

# How does a nursing/breastfeeding mother obtain enough nourishment?

Follow the Wellness Action Plan in Section 1. As a breastfeeding or nursing mother, you need to maintain your energy levels and three proper meals a day and the odd healthy snack will ensure this. Expect to be hungry, but make sure you eat quality, wholesome food and never forget that what you eat goes to your baby too. Why not give both of you the best! Keep up all the nutritional supplements taken during pregnancy, but increase your intake of vitamin C, minerals and essential fatty acid to the following:

- 1 gm vitamin C twice a day

- 2 doses of liquid minerals per day

- 3 capsules of Omega 3 and Omega 6 one of each three times a day with meals

- Otherwise keep to the basic protocol as described in Step 1

- Eat vegetables such as cauliflower, broccoli and cabbage so that your baby does not need a vitamin K injection, which is normally given and is unnecessary in most cases.

## What do I need to know to give my baby the best bonding and attachment?

Early care of the baby actually shapes the developing nervous system and determines what the normal levels of stress are. This is then a base setting for the rest of the baby's adult life.

Touching, stroking, feeding and rocking are all vital. How a mother looks at her baby and her smile and pleasure in caring for him or her will help develop the human part of the brain (the orbitofrontal cortex). This part of the brain in severely neglected babies does not develop properly.

Baby massage is of great benefit. Use light strokes covering the back, down the legs and arms and then repeated on the front. If you want to use a massage oil, it is best to use a cold pressed almond oil.

Good nutrition is vital for the mother and the baby, the quality of the mother's milk depends on her own intake of food, water and nutritional supplements. Apply the Wellness Action Plan Programme in every way.

# *Are there any special check-ups I should give my baby after the birth?*

Paediatric osteopathy is the most superior form of assessment and treatment of your baby's health. Any birth trauma can be released by this approach. Personally, I have had incredible results especially with my twin babies where they had been squashed together in the womb. Any long term compression that may have resulted from this was dealt with miraculously. Once again, prevention paid off!

# *Give me a quick recap on clothes and products that the baby needs.*

Keep it simple. Have plenty of cotton vests, baby grows, 2 or 3 cardigans and nappies/diapers (either reusable or chemically safe ones). All-in-one suits are ideal for outside. How you dress your baby is a personal affair but do bear in mind, for the skin to function properly, the baby's skin needs fabrics that breathe such as cotton and wool. Avoid totally synthetic fabrics as much as possible and always use cotton next to the skin.

Wash your baby's bottom with water and cotton wool to begin with and then use a liquid soap that is free of toxic ingredients as discussed in the Wellness Action Plan step. Avoid using strong perfumes and air fresheners that can harm your baby's delicate nasal passages. Refrain from smothering their skin with baby preparations made from mineral and refined oils. Remember if you can't eat it, don't use it!

# *Tell me about vaccinations.*

Many women have come to me distraught about vaccinations. Media coverage hints from time to time of the dangers and then a few days later there is the counter argument saying that vaccinations are absolutely safe. When discussing it at some doctor's surgeries, mothers are told: "Your child's life is at stake." And "What sort of parent are you to question this?"

We also have to remember that medical school teaches the vaccination programmes to be one of the greatest legacies that modern medicine has given the world. Add the fact that in the UK doctors are only paid when the majority of the children in their practice are vaccinated, so you can see the dilemmas.

Vaccines contain fillers that are known to be toxic to the body. When this is given to a child that is running a temperature and fighting an infection and lacking in minerals and essential fatty acids, you may well have a problem on your hands.

A recent article in the "What Doctors Don't Tell You" newsletter had the headline: "VACCINATIONS: When will parents be told the truth about their safety?" Studies show that side effects or negative reactions are suppressed. And now a new vaccine, PCV, has been brought in to protect against pneumococcalmeningitis, septicaemia and pneumonia. The public is being told the vaccine is safe, but according to WDDTY, they report a study that discovered 117 children have died from the vaccine in Canada where it has been used for the last two years and a further 4,000 children encountered serious reactions.

So what do we do, you may ask? I suggest you look at homeopathic protocols from Ainsworth or Helios to boost the immune system and either use the homeopathic version of the vaccine or use an antidote when you have had the vaccine from your doctor. Make sure your child is well before having a conventional vaccine and supplement his or her diet with a mineral and essential fatty acid supplement. For further reading look at The Vaccination Bible and What The Government Doesn't Tell You About the MMR Vaccine by WDDTY (what doctors don't tell you).

From a holistic point of view, childhood diseases such as measles, mumps and rubella, actually strengthen the immune system and provided they are treated by a holistic practitioner, they will not give long term damage. On the contrary, the child will be stronger as a result.

# What nappies/diapers should I use?

Bringing up a baby is always hectic, so there are times when disposables seem the quickest, easiest nappy solution. However, parents are increasingly concerned about the unregulated chemicals used in disposables.

Most disposable nappies/diapers contain artificial chemical absorbents such as sodium polyacrylate. These chemical granules are used to increase absorbency and form a gel that can end up on your baby as well as in the soil.

Independent US research has also shown that the chemicals in non-cloth disposables can trigger asthma like reactions in normal laboratory animals (US Archives of Environmental Health, October 1999).

Tushies are a cloth-based disposable nappy. With its unique natural cotton blend construction, Tushies offers parents a more reassuring choice, all the performance and ease they expect from a disposable but without the gel.

Green Baby washable nappies/diapers are superb for babies with sensitive skin or ones prone to allergies. Organic cotton is the purest nappy option. As well as organic nappies/diapers, organic muslin squares are available for use as booster pads.

Imse Vimse are a high quality, environmental, award winning cotton flannelette nappy system from Sweden made from certified chemical-free cloth, a great range for babies with sensitive skin. Quick drying, this system is particularly suitable for parents who don't use an automatic dryer.

# How do I start weaning my baby?

The longer a baby is breastfed, the better. The main focus is on the mother looking after herself, eating and drinking plenty of water and taking a rest each day not sitting in front of the TV but lying down either in bed, on the sofa, or even on the floor. When you take a rest like this you can literally feel the breasts filling up with milk! The guidelines for weaning are watching out for the first tooth, a sudden growth spurt where the baby is not satisfied by increased demand feeding, or arriving at the six-month milestone.

The first foods to introduce are fresh, ripe fruits and vegetable purees. The slower these are introduced, the better. This way the baby's digestive system gradually becomes used to breaking down food so there is less likelihood of developing intolerances or the baby being sick. The first tastes are introduced after the milk feed at either the morning or afternoon feed. It is literally a tiny taste. It can be a bit of ripe pear or banana or it can be a taste of pureed organic carrots. Repeat this for 5 days and then introduce another taste. By introducing foods in this way, you can see whether there is any negative reaction or not. Then start two foods a day and little by little you offer more foods. Keep the food smooth as the baby is not able to chew anything yet. However, they do like dry rice cakes to hold and play with. Do not introduce grains until the back molars are in. The reason for this is that the body does not develop the enzymes necessary to break down these types of foods until these teeth are in.

# *Conclusion*

Isn't it amazing how many adults make a rational choice about choosing a partner for life which all too often ends in separation or divorce? Yet when it comes to children, we have no option. We can't give them back and the relationship is there forever. In the end, it makes no difference at what age they walk or talk, they all grow into adults. Survival of the human race continues. So this is a journey that once started can never stop. So we might as well make it as happy and as easy as possible with the thought in mind: to do and be the best possible for all concerned.

So much suffering and misery can be avoided with knowledge and understanding and this is one of the primary purposes of this book.

## *Summary*

By following the Wellness Action Plan and the subsequent steps, there is a far greater chance of gaining wonderful advantages in pregnancy leading to a wonderful birth for both mother and baby, with lasting benefits that go far into adulthood. It is a "win-win" situation.

# The Benefits of following
# Wellness Our Birthright

| For the Mother |
| --- |
| • Improved levels of health as a result of applying the Wellness protocols; |
| • Easier conception; |
| • More enjoyable and healthier pregnancy: avoidance of morning sickness, stretch marks, excessive weight gain, low energy and back problems; |
| • The lasting ability to use her mind in a positive way; |
| • Happier emotional life; |
| • Ability to regain her figure more quickly with no long term damage to any part of her body; |
| • No depression after the baby is born; |
| • Ability to bond effectively with the baby and enjoyment of breastfeeding and caring for a newborn; |
| • More stamina; |
| • Better able to embark on the journey into motherhood. |

| For the New Baby |
|---|
| • Born at term (a full nine months) at ideal weight; |
| • Avoidance of breathing difficulties and need for special care immediately after birth; |
| • Higher immunity; |
| • Less chance of birth defects; |
| • More calm, contented and easier to manage; |
| • Brighter and more loving. |

| And, as the baby grows into Childhood |
|---|
| • Less chance of eczema, asthma, allergies and generally better health; |
| • Better co-ordination including less likelihood of learning and behavioural disabilities such as autism, dyslexia, dyspraxia, ADHD (Attention Deficit Hyperactivity Disorder), Asperger's syndrome; |
| • Higher IQ levels, brighter in general; |
| • Retains higher immunity; |
| • More loving and affectionate. |

| ... And then to Adulthood |
|---|
| • Generally higher levels of healthiness with more emotional stability and the ability to cope better with life's inevitable challenges; |
| • Well formed brain; |
| • Brighter adult; |
| • Reduced chances of having diseases later on in life such as heart and cardiovascular problems, cancers and diabetes; |
| • Better reproductive health, whether male or female; |
| • All body systems start at a higher level: hormonal, digestive and immune systems. |

*Over to You*

# Over to You

Now you know that parents who have an understanding of the long term consequences of preparation for pre-pregnancy, pregnancy, childbirth and breastfeeding are more likely to have healthier, happier children with less addictive and behavioural problems, for example, drug addiction, schizophrenia, anorexia, autism, dyslexia and dyspraxia and even suicide. The children will have fewer chances of birth defects and of developing eczema, asthma and allergies due to stronger immune systems with reduced chances of disease and even cancers later on in life. So much can be prevented with understanding and an action plan.

If medical intervention is needed as an emergency rescue, then so be it. The woman, in this instance, should not see that she has failed in her attempt to experience a natural pregnancy and birth. Rather, she did everything she could and has been wise in knowing when to ask for help. Most importantly, she will still be able to give her infant the best possible care now that she has read this book.

No one person can define love. Perhaps the ultimate form of love among humans might be the love of Nature or, in other words, a great respect for Mother Earth. The first hour of life is a critical period and, together with the emotional welcome and physical contact from the mother, will determine the baby's level of respect and ability to love human kind in general. When the birth process comes to be seen, in particular by health professionals, as an episode of sexual life and as a critical period in the development of our capacity to love, the human race may move on to another level of evolution.

In the words of Deepak Chopra, MD, one of the most important healers of our time:

> "If every mother could create a covenant with her baby, the whole world would be transformed. Every terrorist was once a baby and so was every saint. The world hangs precariously in the choices made by mothers."

> "The world was never changed or transformed by politicians, or for that matter, by scientists. The mothers of the world hold the key to the healing of our wounded planet."

*Wellness Our Birthright* has been written to help give women faith in their bodies, to guide women to open their hearts and let go of their minds and to encourage them to put the love back into childbirth.

Who can make a difference in this world? **You**, yes you! You can share this information with others and so reduce some of the needless suffering that is caused by lack of knowledge and wisdom. This way, we can help raise happier, healthier children not only for this generation but for those to come so that Wellness is indeed their birthright. What greater legacy can a parent give their child?

# *Index of Questions*

## *Step 3 – Pregnancy*    *93*

## Step 4 – Birth                                                129

# Recommended Reading

*Birthing from Within, An extraordinary Guide to Childbirth Preparation:* Pam England and Rob Horowitz

*Birth and Breastfeeding:* Michel Odent

*Breaking through Limitations:* John Kanary

*Holistic Guide To Pregnancy And Childbirth:* Deepak Chopra, MD

*Immaculate Deception I I:* Suzanne Arms

*Ina May's Guide to Childbirth:* Ina May Gaskin

*Not on the Label:* Felicity Lawrence

*Shopped: The Shocking Powers of British Supermarkets:* Joanna Blythman

*Stop the 21st Century Killing You:* Dr Paula Baillie-Hamilton

*The Thinking Woman's Guide to a Better Birth:* Henci Goer

*The Scientification of Love:* Michel Odent

*Unreasonable Risk:* Samual S Epstein, MD

*You Can Heal Your Life:* Louise L Hay

*Why Love Matters:* Sue Gerhardt

# Bibliography

Ballentine MD, Rudolph. *Diet And Nutrition.* Honesdale, Pennsylvania: The Himalayan International Institute. 1979

Baillie-Hamilton, Dr. Paula. *Stop The 21st Century Killing You.* London: The Vermilon. 2005

Balaskas, Janet. *Active Birth.* London: Unwin Paperbacks. 1993

Batmanghelidj, Dr. F. *Your Body's Many Cries For Water.* London: The Therapist. 1997

Blackmore, M C H. *Mineral Deficiencies In Human Cells.* Sydney: Blackmores Communications Service. 1983

Blythman, Joanna. *Shopped, The Shocking Powers Of British Supermarkets.* London: Harper Perennial. 2005

Brennan, Barbara Ann. *Hands of Light.* New York: Bantan Book. 1988

Brennan, Barbara Ann. *Light Emerging.* New York: Bantan Book. 1993

Chaitow ND, DO, MBNOA. *Relaxation And Medication Techniques.* Wellingborough, England: Thorsons. 1983

Chopra MD, Deepak. *Creating Health.* London: Rider. 2004

Chopra, MD, Deepak. *Holistic Guide To Pregnancy And Childbirth.* New York: Three Rivers Press. 2005

Compiles By Ovulation Method Advisory Service OMAS. *Ovulation Method Billings.* London: Cork Billings NFP Centre.

Covey, Stephen R. *The 7 Habits of Highly Effective People.* Uk: Simon and Schuster UK Ltd. 1992.

Davidson, John and Farida. *Fertility Awareness.* Saffron Walden, England: The C.W. Daniel Company. 1986

Drake, Katia and Jonathan. *Natural Birth Control.* Wellingborough, England: Thorsons Publishers Ltd. 1985

Emoto, Masaru. *The Hidden Messages In Water.* Oregon: Beyond Words Publishing. 2004

Emoto, Masaru. *The True Power of Water.* Oregon: Beyond Words Publishing. 2005

England Cnm, MA, Pam and Horowitz PhD, Bob. *Birthing From Within.* New Mexico: Partera Press. 1998

Epstein MD, Samual S. *Unreasonable Risk.* Chicago: Environmental Toxicology Inc. 2005

Fisher, Leslie. *Clinical Science Of Mineral Therapy.* New South Wales, Australia: The Maurice Blackmore Research Foundation. 1991

Gaskin, Ina May. *Ina May's Guide To Childbirth.* New York: Bantam Dell Random House. 2003

Gerhardt, Sue. *Why Love Matters.* London, New York: Routledge. 2004

Goer, Henci. *The Thinking Woman's Guide To A Better Birth.* New York: Perigee Book. 1999

Gordon, Dr Yehudi. *Birth and Beyond.* London: Vermilion, 2002

Hay, Louise L. *You Can Heal Your Life.* London: Eden Grove Editions. 1984

Herrmann, Christer-Maria. *Movement Of Life In The Five Elements.* Spain: Centreur. 1996

Holford, Patrick and Lawson, Susannah. *Optimum Nutrition, Before, During And After Pregnancy.* London: Piatkus Ltd. 2004

Jacka, P A. *Naturopathic Clinical Medicine.* Australia: Dee Y Printing Works. 1983

Kadans, ND, PHD, Joseph M. *Encyclopedia Of Medicinal Foods.* Wellingborough, England: Thorsonsr Publishers Ltd. 1982

Kellner-Read, Bill. *Toxic Bite.* Tunbridge, England: Credence Publications. 2002

Kitzinger, Sheila. *Breastfeeding Your Baby.* Dorling Kindersley. London. 1989

Kitzinger, Sheila. *The New Pregnancy and Childbirth.* Dorling Kindersley, London. 2003

Lawrence, Felicity. *Not On The Label.* London: Penguin Books. 2004

Lee, Deborah. *Essential Fatty Acids.* Pleasant Grove, UT: Woodland Publishing.

Lyth, Geoff and Charles, Sue. *Aromatherapy Lexicon.* East Horsley, England: Amber Wood Publishing.

Millwood, Dr. John. *The Treason Within.* England: Health Issues Ltd. Bucks. 2005

Motha, Dr. Gowri. *Gentle Birth Method*. London: Thorsons. 2004

Odent, Michel. *Birth and Breastfeeding*. London: Clairview. 2003

Odent, Michel. *Primal Health*. Forest Row, England: Clair View Books. 2002

Odent, Michel. *The Caesarean*. London: Free Association Books. 2004

Odent, Michel. *The Farmer And The Obstetrician*. London: Free Association Books. 2002

Odent, Michel. *The Scientification of Love*. London: Free Association Books. 2001

Pearce, Joseph Chilton. *Magical Child Rediscovering Nature's Plan for our Children*. Joseph Chilton Pearce.

Pert, PhD, Candace B. *Molecules of Emotion*. London, New York, Sidney, Tokyo, and Toronto: Pocket Books, 1999

Price DDS, Weston A, *Nutrition And Physical Degeneration*. C.A.: Pottenger Nutrition Foundation Inc. 1945

Rolls, Prof. Edmund T. *Emotion Explained*. Oxford: Oxford University Press. 2005

Rothera, Ellen. *Allergies In The Under Fives. Environmental Assistance*. Grimsby. 2004

Stern, D, Bruschweiler-Stern, N, Freeland, A *The Birth of a Mother*. London: Bloomsbury Publishing.1998

Supper, Jennie. *The Pregnancy Book*. London: Amberwood Publishing, 1998

Sutton, Jean and Scott, Paulene. *Optimal Foetal Positioning*. Tauranga, NZ: Birth Concepts. 1996

Trattler, Ross. *Better Health Through Natural Healing*. London: Thorsons. 1987

Walker, Dr. N. W. *Vibrant Health*. Phoenix, Arizona: O'Sullivan Woodside & Co. 1983

West, Zita. *Natural Pregnancy*. London: Dorling Kindersley. 2001

Woollams, Chris. *Everything You Need to Know to Help You Beat Cancer*. Buckingham: Health Issues Ltd. 2002

Woollams, Chris. Oestrogen, *The Killer In Our Midst*. Buckingham: Health Issues Ltd. 2004

# *About the Author*

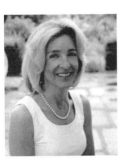

**Vivien Clere Green** is a Natural Health Consultant, Practitioner and Speaker who takes a holistic and integrated approach to health and nutrition. Qualified to practice in a number of different modalities, her training started 26 years ago in Nutrition and Naturopathy (nature cure) and was then followed by Iridology, Shiatsu, Reflexology, Rayid, Homotoxicology and Bio-Regulatory Medicine (modern or complex homeopathy, using the latest European research and development). She is a Registered Member of a number of different organisations, including the Institute of Complementary Medicine.

Her interest in nutrition started at 19 and gradually took over more and more of her life. As a result, she left the financial world of the City to run a whole food business, which opened doors to her becoming a practitioner. She had the good fortune to apprentice to a very gifted Naturopath and Osteopath, John Sugarman, N.D.D.O., who subsequently became her Mentor. He won the Practitioner of the Year Award in 1990 awarded by JACM (Journal of Alternative and Complementary Medicine) and it was he who started her on her path of preparing for pregnancy, natural childbirth and exclusive breastfeeding.

Her work revolves around maintaining optimum health. She specializes in helping women, including those who have difficulty conceiving, prepare for pregnancy and takes them through pregnancy, birth and breastfeeding. In her capacity as a doula she can attend the birth itself. For the last 23 years she has been in practice in England, 15 years in London and 8 years in Oxfordshire. Vivien and her husband, Richard, have five children, all of whom were born naturally, including twins born in her early forties.

The UK's number one charity for complementary therapies and cancer prevention.

For the latest information, breakthroughs and news on cancer prevention and cure, see icon magazine

For a free trial copy -Tel: 44(0)1280 821211

icon  CANCER active

# Wellness Action Plan

"Many of the products discussed earlier in Step 1 are being constantly improved with new ones being introduced all the time. I therefore decided to direct you to my website for the latest updates as well as information on individual and corporate programmes. Plus free enews updates and web links."

www.viviencleregreen.com

info@viviencleregreen.com

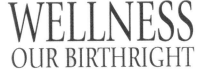

WELLNESS
OUR BIRTHRIGHT

# birthlight

For the Greater Enjoyment of Pregnancy, Birth and Babies

- Prenatal Yoga and YogaCise
- Prenatal AquaYoga
- Birth Preparation
- Waterbirth Preparation
- Postnatal Yoga and YogaCise
- Baby Nurture
- Baby Yoga
- Baby Yoga for Toddlers
- Infant Aquatics
- Well Woman Yoga

Contact: (+44) 01223 362288, www.birthlight.com

Birthlight is a registered charity (No: 1088207)

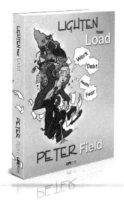

Lighten Your Load

Peter Field

ISBN # 1-59930-000-1

Your Doctor Said WHAT?
Exposing The Communication Gap

Terrie Wurzbacher

ISBN # 1-59930-029-X

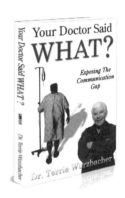

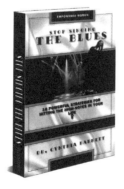

Stop Singing The Blues
10 Powerful Strategies For Hitting The
High Notes In Your Life

Dr Cynthia Barnett

ISBN # 1-59930-022-2

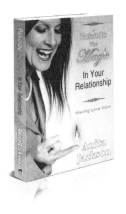

Rekindle The Magic In Your Relationship
Making Love Work

Anita Jackson

ISBN # 1-59930-041-9

Wellness Our Birthright
How to give a baby the best start in life.

Vivien Clere Green

ISBN # 1-59930-020-6

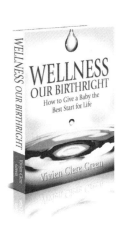

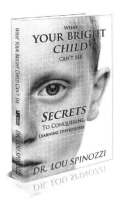

What Your Bright Child Can't See
Secrets To Conquering Learning
Difficulties

Dr Lou Spinozzi

ISBN # 1-59930-033-8